Deluxe Keto & Low Carb Food Journal

By Habitually Healthy Publishing

Your greatest wealth is your health.

Habitually Healthy Publishing offers the information in this journal for informational purposes only and makes no claims regards the interpretation or utilization of any information in the journal.

All rights are reserved, including the right to reproduce this journal in whole, or any portion, in any form.

www.habitually-healthy.com

> **"STRIVE FOR PROGRESS NOT PERFECTION."**

DEDICATION

This journal is dedicated to you.
For taking the first small step and deciding to be just that little bit better.

CONTENTS

Introduction 6
- Why Journaling Works 8
- Journal Overview 10
- Four-Step Plan for Your Success 10
- Making Keto easier, faster and more effective – online guides 12

Step 1 – Setting intentions 14
- Personal Goals 15
- Daily Food Targets 17

Step 2 – Tracking Food 20
- Weekly Preparation 21
- How This Book Works 22
- Notes on Completing the Diary 26
- Daily Tracking
    - Month 1 30
    - Month 2 98
    - Month 3 162

Step 3 – Review 225
- Before and After 226
- Tracking Charts 228
- Weekly Progress Chart 229

Contents

Step 4 - Celebrate **236**
- 3-Month Target Achieved 237

Appendix **239**
- Calories Burned by Exercise – Reference 240
- Frequently Eaten Foods 242
- Recipe Notes 244

INTRODUCTION

> A study of nearly 1,700 participants shows that keeping a food diary can double a person's weight-loss[1].
> —*Kaiser Permanente's Center for Health Research*

We have often read forums, spoken with friends, and received emails from people on a ketogenic or low-carbohydrate diet stating they lost weight but struggled with maintaining their *discipline or breaking through plateaus*. We knew the traditional advice wasn't enough. "Try harder," "eat fewer calories," "exercise more," "try raspberry ketones," and so on was either outdated, did not work, or was just not helpful.

We started to look at the science behind motivation, discipline, and weight loss. Through our research, it became clear that a journal would be the answer. However, we did not want to create just "another way to track calories," we wanted to create a journal to support you fully.

ROUND PEGS AND SQUARE HOLES
Trying to use a normal food diary on the ketogenic or low-carb diet is like trying to put a round peg in a square hole.

It just doesn't fit. The design of generic food journals is typically created for a standard American diet with conventional advice for general health, such as eating lots of slow-release carbs, whole grains, fruits, and so on. With this in mind, we realized that, although all the information we need to start a ketogenic diet is already at our fingertips, we are missing one vital tool: a journal that caters specifically to the ketogenic diet and lifestyle.

---
[1] https://www.sciencedaily.com/releases/2008/07/080708080738.htm

Introduction

This was our inspiration in creating the keto/low-carb journal. A beautifully crafted planner, tailored specifically for you on your keto or low-carb diet journey. It includes the key component measures of ketogenic dieting and all the advice and encouragement you will need on your journey.

NOT JUST A FOOD JOURNAL
We looked at the science of motivation and included the best tools and strategies to ensure you are motivated and keep progressing toward your health goals.

By supporting you in your progression and recording your daily food intake and exercise routine, the accountability and practice of writing everything down will help motivate you to focus on and achieve your goals. You will be inspired to remain disciplined and maintain good habits.

While the journal is tailored for the keto diet, please feel free to use as much or as little of the diary as you like. It is designed to be flexible depending on your goals and preferences. Our goal was to design an appealing and accessible product, created specifically to meet your needs.

Weight-loss success takes keeping track of everything you are putting in your body, having a plan and implementing it, and using the science of motivation – not just willpower – to achieve your goals daily.

That's where this journal completes the puzzle. Use this diary alongside a ketogenic or low-carb diet and you will double your chances of succeeding. Whether you are just starting a diet, trying to break through a plateau, or just want to try something different, you will surely find the help you need in these pages.

WHY JOURNALING WORKS

Researchers (and marketers) have known for a long time that the majority of our decisions are subconscious. One study concludes that "your brain makes up its mind up to 10 seconds before you realize it."[2] Unfortunately, our unconscious decisions tend not to be what is best for us.

When you see that chocolate donut, your brain has already decided it wants it and it is very hard to fight that impulse.

We need to take our (negative) eating and exercising habits off autopilot and be aware of our decision making. We can then rewire our brain to make the positive habits our new autopilot. This is the power of a journal.

Simply having a journal makes us aware of our habits by:

- Creating awareness of current eating patterns
- Offering accountability to yourself for your goals
- Establishing new positive habits
- Keeping you motivated with tangible, documented, and positive results from your efforts.

---

[2] https://www.relationshipscoach.co.uk/blog/research-shows-our-subconscious-mind-makes-our-decisions-for-us/

> **"THERE IS NO ONE GIANT STEP THAT DOES IT. IT'S LOTS OF LITTLE STEPS"**

JOURNAL OVERVIEW

FOUR-STEP PLAN FOR YOUR SUCCESS

Step 1: Set Goals – Create Motivation
Setting realistic goals and stating why you want to achieve them will help you get started and keep going when it gets tough.

Step 2: Take Action – Write It Down
Track your food, beverage, and exercise regimen so you stay disciplined and accountable for your goals. Aside from just recording your food, reaffirming your goals, reviewing the previous week and motivational quotes help to keep you on track.

Step 3: Review Your Progress
Check your progress periodically and take pride in your accomplishments to reinforce your new positive eating habits. In this section you will find ways to:

- Record your before and after measurements
- Visually track your progress on line charts (using any measurement you want)

Step 4: Celebrate
Commemorate all the small and big wins so you can stay motivated and continue moving toward your goals.

Making Keto Easier, Faster, and More Effective – Online downloadable guides
Inside this section are invaluable guides that will make your ketogenic lifestyle easier. Learn how to overcome plateaus, use intermittent fasting for greater fat burning, and get into ketosis quicker than ever. Want to know the best day to start a diet (according to science), you'll find that here too.

Appendix

This section includes an abundance of useful information and a place for your own notes. It contains a

- guide to calories burned by common exercise.
- pages to record your most frequent food nutritional information.
- store your favorite keto recipes.

MAKING KETO EASIER, FASTER AND MORE EFFECTIVE ONLINE GUIDES

This an online section intended to make your lifestyle on a keto diet that little much easier and overcoming some key challenges you might find along the way, from dealing with keto flu to overcoming plateaus to "tricking" yourself into losing more weight – all backed by science.

These are intended to be "extras" and are not essential for a ketogenic diet. We would recommend having a read and see if any ideas jump out at you or come back to this section if you are having a specific problem, such as having reached a plateau.

Visit the below site to download your guide.

www.habitually-healthy.com/hacks

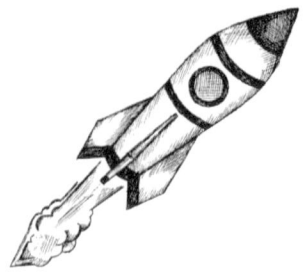

Bonus Fat Bombs & Desserts ebook

Thank you for purchasing the deluxe food journal. To provide you with some scumptious recipes, we asked keto chef extraordinaire, Elizabeth Jane, for a little help.

She provides 20 of her favorite fat-burning sweet and savory treats.

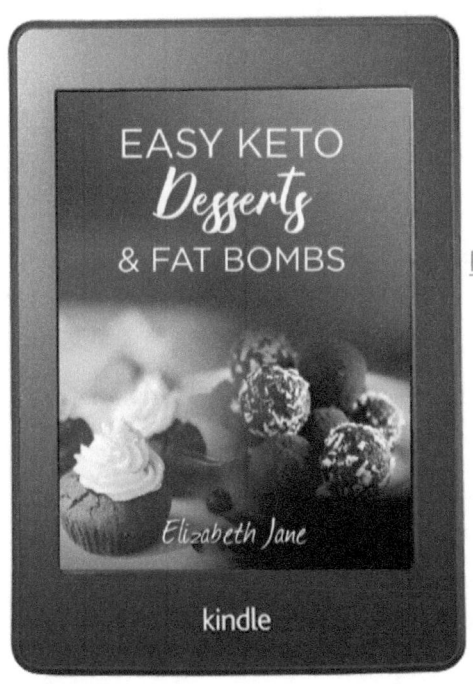

To download simply visit

http://habitually-healthy.com/bombs

No sign ups or email address needed, just downloaded your delectable keto snacks now.

STEP 1
SETTING INTENTIONS

Simply writing your food down is not enough. Prepare and motivate yourself and take the 7-day challenge to keep on track.

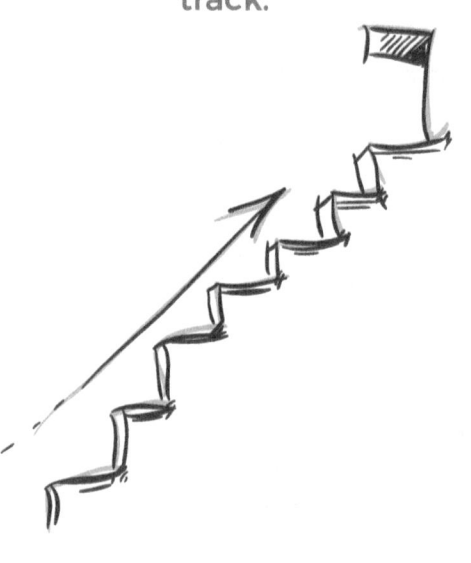

Step 1 – Setting Intentions

PERSONAL GOALS

"(S)he who has a why to live for can bear almost anyhow."
— *Friedrich Nietzsche*

Having a goal and a strong "why" will keep you motivated when it gets hard.

The goal doesn't have to be to lose X amount of pounds. It could be instead simply to complete three months of the diary. What is of *greater importance is your "why"* – your reason for wanting to achieve the goal.

Wanting to lose weight just for the sake of losing weight is not usually motivating enough. You may wish to lose weight for health reasons, to be able to play with your new nephew, to attend a wedding that is coming up, or perhaps to feel more confident in yourself. There may be a small reward involved like a vacation, massage, or some new clothes.

It is your reason that will keep you motivated. Make sure it is strong.

Goal:_____

_____

I will achieve this by:

_____

I will achieve this because:

_____

_____

_____

_____

TIPS FOR GOAL SETTING

- **Make it specific.** For example, if you want to lose weight, write, "Lose 10 pounds within next 4 weeks." If you are working specifically on your physique, write "Lose 2 inches in the next six weeks."
- **Use the affirmative.** Rather than "I want to lose 10 pounds," write "I will lose 10 pounds ...." Such statements have proven to have subtle positive effects on your mind.
- **Make it realistic.** Losing 50 pounds in a week is not reasonable and will lead to disappointment. Make it a "Goldilocks" goal – not too easy and not too hard.
- **Set a deadline.** Having an end point of time involved makes the goal more real. This journal is for three months, so consider that as a deadline.

THREE MONTHS FROM NOW, YOU WILL THANK YOURSELF.

DAILY FOOD TARGETS

Record your daily targets for food and exercise.

Calculating your targets can be complicated, particularly if taking into account variables, such as age, gender, daily activity, and so on. I would recommend using the calculator at ruled.me, which considers a range of factors including your lifestyle and weight-loss targets.

https://www.ruled.me/keto-calculator/

Revisit this calculator monthly. If you lose weight, your targets will change accordingly.

Calories:_____ Fats:_____ Carbs:_____

Net Carbs:_____ Protein:_____

Not everyone needs to go to the gym to get the benefits of exercise. One study claims walking just 20 minutes a day cuts your risk of premature death by almost one-third.[3]

Physical activity target

Week:_____

Day:_____

Quantity / Time:_____

See the end of the book for a "calories burned by exercise" reference guide.

---

[3] http://www.cam.ac.uk/research/news/lack-of-exercise-responsible-for-twice-as-many-deaths-as-obesity

7-DAY CHALLENGE

I am confident that if you can complete this diary for just seven days, then you can complete it for 14 days. If you can complete 14 days, then you can complete 30 days. After 30 days, you can then go on to 60 days and then 90 days.

If you can complete 90 days, then you will have achieved almost any health goal you have set.

The first seven days are the hardest, but we have a few tools to keep you going. In this book, you will find sections that:

- **Motivate you** – Set your intentions with your goals and reasons why
- **Keep you disciplined** – Set daily targets to stay on track
- **Inspire you** – Make some dishes from recipe ideas that make you feel creative. Find our favorite places to find recipes in the downloadable guide.
- **Make it fun** – This journal has been designed to make your transition into the keto lifestyle a fun process

THE CHALLENGE

If you can do these simple tasks every day for seven days, you will be well on your way to achieving your goals:

1. **Review your goals and reasons every morning.** – Keep yourself motivated and keep your goals in mind.
2. **Take your diary (and pen) everywhere you go.** – Hold yourself accountable everywhere with this journal.
3. **Write everything down.** Fill in this diary anytime you eat or drink something immediately when you consume it.
4. **Review it at the end of every day.** Review your accomplishments each day and celebrate every step closer to your goals.
5. **Celebrate on day seven.** At the end of the week, celebrate that you completed the challenge (fat bombs are particularly good for this).

This entire process should take you no longer than 30 minutes every day. That is 3½ hours out of 168 in your entire week (or 2 percent of your time). It takes just a small-time commitment to achieve your big goals.

STEP 2
TRACKING FOOD

This is where 'the rubber meets the road', and you put in the hard work to track your food intake.

You'll also find best practices, motivation and celebrations in the section to help you on your journey.

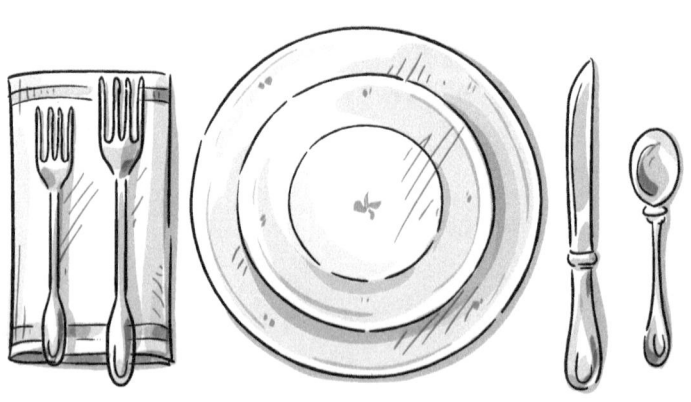

WEEKLY PREPARATION

MAKING DECISIONS THE EASY WAY

In the report 'What You Need To Know About Willpower: The Psychological Science of Self-control',[4] the American Psychological Association states "A growing body of research shows that resisting repeated temptations takes a mental toll." Some experts liken willpower to a muscle that can get fatigued from overuse.

This is similar to gas in a tank, the more decisions you make during a day, the more decision fatigued you become. Rest and recuperation then replenishes your tank. This explains why you are more likely to break a diet towards the end of the day than the start of a day.

HOW TO STAY ON TRACK WHEN DECISION MAKING FATIGUE OCCURS

As your day progresses, your "tank" will deplete, and you will begin to make habitual decisions, which at the start will likely be non-keto food (whatever is closest to hand).

Plan out your days and weeks in advance and "make the decision" ahead of time. Plan your meals and get snacks ready.

Attempt to establish a habit of planning and preparing meals either on the weekend or the night before and your chances of success will increase further.

---

[4] http://www.apa.org/helpcenter/willpower.aspx

HOW THIS BOOK WORKS - RECORDING FOOD

Over the next few pages, the daily food log will be introduced, with explanations and examples of how to use each section.

1 Date and Day - Circle the day and enter the date. Include a day number if you wish.

2 Food Tracking - Contains all of the required details for a ketogenic diet. If possible, try and plan it out the day before – this will help to resist urges for "convenient snacks." Enter the time of the food, which can help with intermittent fasting and to notice trends.

3 Water - Try to consume the recommended eight 8-ounce glasses of water. Cross them out as you drink each glass.

Step 2 – Tracking Food

Date: Day 1 – 1st January   Mon. Tue. Wed. Thur. Fri. (Sat.) Sun.

BREAKFAST	Amount	Cal.	Fat gm	Carb. gm	Fiber gm	Net Carb. gm	Protein gm
Zucchini	½	16	0	3	1	2	1
Salmon fillet	1 fillet	241	14				28
Green onions	½ cup	16	0	2	2		
Coconut oil	1 tbsp	120	14				
Crumbled feta	½ cup	198	16	3		3	10
⊙ midday TOTAL		591	44	8	3	5	39

SNACK	Amount	Cal.	Fat gm	Carb. gm	Fiber gm	Net Carb. gm	Protein gm
Bulletproof coffee	1 cup	228	26				
⊙ 2pm TOTAL							

LUNCH	Amount	Cal.	Fat gm	Carb. gm	Fiber gm	Net Carb. gm	Protein gm
Pesto Spaghetti	1 serve	521	45	2	1	1	29
⊙ 3pm TOTAL							

SNACK	Amount	Cal.	Fat gm	Carb. gm	Fiber gm	Net Carb. gm	Protein gm
Hummus + cucumber	50g	125	9	5	2	3	5
⊙ 6pm TOTAL							

✘ ✘ ✘ ✘ ▢ ▢ ▢ ▢   8 oz

4 Daily Total and Target - Sum your daily total calories and macronutrients. You may not require them all – such as fiber.

Daily target - Enter your daily targets for calories and macronutrients. Compare them to your actual totals at the end of the day. How close were they?

5 Ketone Levels - This gauge is for recording your ketone levels. Visually, it indicates whether you are in ketosis (0-5-3.0mm) within the large markers. Mark off and record your levels. There is also a daily tracking chart in the reference section for a visual record over time.

6 Recording Exercise - Recording even the smallest exercise is beneficial as it shows your improvement and is motivating to reflect on. In the reference section is a guide to calories burned by common exercises.

7 Fasting Clock - If you are fasting, record the time your fast began and finished to calculate the number of hours fasted. This is a daily tracking chart in the reference section – again for a visual record over time.

8 Vitamins, Supplements, and Medications- List any supplements or medicine you are taking. This can be useful as a reminder or as a record to look back on later.

9 How was today - Record small wins, how you felt, and what you might do better tomorrow (set a positive intent).

Step 2 – Tracking Food

DINNER	Amount	Cal.	Fat gm	Carb. gm	Fiber gm	Net Carb. gm	Protein gm
chicken breast	1	231	5				43
avocado	½ med	70	7	4	1	3	
Pesto - homemade!	2 tsp	12	1				
⏱ 7pm TOTAL		313	13	4	1	3	43

SNACK	Amount	Cal.	Fat gm	Carb. gm	Fiber gm	Net Carb. gm	Protein gm
⏱ 8pm TOTAL							

| Daily Total | | 1613 | 128 | 14 | 5 | 9 | 11 |
| Daily Target | | 1500 | 133 | 20 | | 20 | 58 |

Ketone Levels (mM): 2.4 (X marked between 2.0 and 3.0)
Scale: 0 0.5 1.0 1.5 2.0 3.0 5.0+

Fasting Clock
Fast start: 8pm yesterday
Fast finish: midday
Hours fasted: 14 hrs

Exercise notes
What: walked to store
Duration: 30 mins
Calories Burned: 160

Vitamins / Supplements / Meds.

Description	Qty	
Potassium	1	1
Multi vitamin	1	

How was today?
Over keto flu (yay!). Felt good today. Macros were good (bit too much protein... will watch it tomorrow. Overall happy with day!

😞 😔 😐 🙂 **😄** (last emoji circled)

NOTES ON COMPLETING THE DIARY

- **Don't skip the front section.** The "Personal Goals" section will help keep you motivated so you can maintain your discipline.
- **Be as accurate as possible.** It is easy to try and "guess" portions. Try to record it when you consume it.
- **Include all the extras.** That coffee you picked up while you were out or that little nibble on a fat bomb – they all count! Write it down.
- **Don't beat yourself up over mistakes.** Know that you will slip up but don't give yourself a hard time. Write it down and learn from it moving forward.
- **Review your diary.** Reviewing your diary on a weekly basis will reveal progression and eating patterns, which will help to keep you motivated.
- **Keep it with you, everywhere.** Recording your food and drink "in the moment" is always more preferable than trying to remember something later. We tend to forget or distort what we actually consumed. It's best to write it down immediately so you don't have to rely on your memory.
- **Be as detailed as you want to be.** This diary provides all the information you could need but it should feel easy and not like a chore when completing the meals.
- **Cook at home.** Try cooking at home as much as possible, as it makes recording your food that much easier.
- **Connect with the tracking.** Try not to 'just write' your food down, but get a 'sense' for what 400 calories or you total daily calorie count physically looks like. It will help you feel how much food you need to 'be full'. This is intuitive eating and could mean no longer tracking food (if you wish).

REAFFIRMING COMMITMENT

Studies have shown "you become 42% more likely to achieve your goals and dreams, simply by writing them down on a regular basis".[5]

It is the start of a new week, so reaffirm your commitment to your goals and increase your chances of success. When writing your goals 'feel' they are coming true and ensure your reasons for wanting the goal are strong.

Goal:_____

_____

I will achieve this by:

_____

I will achieve this because:

_____
_____
_____
_____

---

[5] https://www.huffingtonpost.com/marymorrissey/the-power-of-writing-down_b_12002348.html

NOW IT IS YOUR TURN.

Focus on the single step / day in front of you.

Before starting your first day, remember:

Decide

Commit

Prepare

Take consistent positive action

> "YOU DO NOT HAVE TO SEE **THE WHOLE STAIRCASE,** JUST TAKE THE **FIRST STEP**"

WEEK OF ___

Date: _____ Mon. Tue. Wed. Thur. Fri. Sat. Sun.

BREAKFAST	Amount	Cal.	Fat gm	Carb. gm	Fiber gm	Net Carb. gm	Protein gm
TOTAL							

SNACK	Amount	Cal.	Fat gm	Carb. gm	Fiber gm	Net Carb. gm	Protein gm
TOTAL							

LUNCH	Amount	Cal.	Fat gm	Carb. gm	Fiber gm	Net Carb. gm	Protein gm
TOTAL							

SNACK	Amount	Cal.	Fat gm	Carb. gm	Fiber gm	Net Carb. gm	Protein gm
TOTAL							

8 oz

Step 2 – Tracking Food

DINNER	Amount	Cal.	Fat gm	Carb. gm	Fiber gm	Net Carb. gm	Protein gm
🕒 TOTAL							

SNACK	Amount	Cal.	Fat gm	Carb. gm	Fiber gm	Net Carb. gm	Protein gm
🕒 TOTAL							
Daily Total							
Daily Target							

Ketone Levels (mM)

0   0.5   1.0   1.5   2.0   2.5   3.0   5.0+

Fasting Clock
Fast start _____   Hours fasted
Fast finish _____

Exercise notes
What _____
Duration _____
Calories Burned _____

Vitamins / Supplements / Meds.

Description	Qty

How was today?

_____

_____

DAILY

Date: _____   Mon. Tue. Wed. Thur. Fri. Sat. Sun.

BREAKFAST	Amount	Cal.	Fat gm	Carb. gm	Fiber gm	Net Carb. gm	Protein gm
🕐 TOTAL							

SNACK	Amount	Cal.	Fat gm	Carb. gm	Fiber gm	Net Carb. gm	Protein gm
🕐 TOTAL							

LUNCH	Amount	Cal.	Fat gm	Carb. gm	Fiber gm	Net Carb. gm	Protein gm
🕐 TOTAL							

SNACK	Amount	Cal.	Fat gm	Carb. gm	Fiber gm	Net Carb. gm	Protein gm
🕐 TOTAL							

8 oz

Step 2 – Tracking Food

DINNER	Amount	Cal.	Fat gm	Carb. gm	Fiber gm	Net Carb. gm	Protein gm
⏲ TOTAL							

SNACK	Amount	Cal.	Fat gm	Carb. gm	Fiber gm	Net Carb. gm	Protein gm
⏲ TOTAL							
Daily Total							
Daily Target							

Ketone Levels (mM)

|—|—|—|—|—|—|—|—|—|—|
0   0.5 1.0 1.5 2.0 2.5 3.0   5.0+

Fasting Clock

Fast start _____   Hours fasted [   ]

Fast finish _____

Exercise notes

What _____

Duration _____

Calories Burned _____

Vitamins / Supplements / Meds.

Description	Qty

How was today?

_____

_____

DAILY

Date: _____   Mon. Tue. Wed. Thur. Fri. Sat. Sun.

BREAKFAST	Amount	Cal.	Fat gm	Carb. gm	Fiber gm	Net Carb. gm	Protein gm
🕐 TOTAL							

SNACK	Amount	Cal.	Fat gm	Carb. gm	Fiber gm	Net Carb. gm	Protein gm
🕐 TOTAL							

LUNCH	Amount	Cal.	Fat gm	Carb. gm	Fiber gm	Net Carb. gm	Protein gm
🕐 TOTAL							

SNACK	Amount	Cal.	Fat gm	Carb. gm	Fiber gm	Net Carb. gm	Protein gm
🕐 TOTAL							

8 oz

Step 2 – Tracking Food

DINNER	Amount	Cal.	Fat gm	Carb. gm	Fiber gm	Net Carb. gm	Protein gm
TOTAL							

SNACK	Amount	Cal.	Fat gm	Carb. gm	Fiber gm	Net Carb. gm	Protein gm
TOTAL							

| Daily Total | | | | | | | |
| Daily Target | | | | | | | |

Ketone Levels (mM)

0   0.5   1.0   1.5   2.0   2.5   3.0   5.0+

Fasting Clock

Fast start _____

Fast finish _____

Hours fasted

Exercise notes

What _____

Duration _____

Calories Burned _____

Vitamins / Supplements / Meds.

Description	Qty

How was today?

_____

_____

DAILY

Date: _____   Mon. Tue. Wed. Thur. Fri. Sat. Sun.

BREAKFAST	Amount	Cal.	Fat gm	Carb. gm	Fiber gm	Net Carb. gm	Protein gm
🕐 TOTAL							

SNACK	Amount	Cal.	Fat gm	Carb. gm	Fiber gm	Net Carb. gm	Protein gm
🕐 TOTAL							

LUNCH	Amount	Cal.	Fat gm	Carb. gm	Fiber gm	Net Carb. gm	Protein gm
🕐 TOTAL							

SNACK	Amount	Cal.	Fat gm	Carb. gm	Fiber gm	Net Carb. gm	Protein gm
🕐 TOTAL							

8 oz

Step 2 – Tracking Food

DINNER	Amount	Cal.	Fat gm	Carb. gm	Fiber gm	Net Carb. gm	Protein gm
⊘ _____ TOTAL							

SNACK	Amount	Cal.	Fat gm	Carb. gm	Fiber gm	Net Carb. gm	Protein gm
⊘ _____ TOTAL							
Daily Total							
Daily Target							

Ketone Levels (mM)
0   0.5   1.0   1.5   2.0   2.5   3.0   5.0+

Fasting Clock
Fast start _____
Fast finish _____
Hours fasted ☐

Exercise notes
What _____
Duration _____
Calories Burned _____

Vitamins / Supplements / Meds.

Description	Qty

How was today?
_____
_____

DAILY

Date: Mon.   Tue.   Wed.   Thur.   Fri.   Sat.   Sun.

BREAKFAST	Amount	Cal.	Fat gm	Carb. gm	Fiber gm	Net Carb. gm	Protein gm
🕐 TOTAL							

SNACK	Amount	Cal.	Fat gm	Carb. gm	Fiber gm	Net Carb. gm	Protein gm
🕐 TOTAL							

LUNCH	Amount	Cal.	Fat gm	Carb. gm	Fiber gm	Net Carb. gm	Protein gm
🕐 TOTAL							

SNACK	Amount	Cal.	Fat gm	Carb. gm	Fiber gm	Net Carb. gm	Protein gm
🕐 TOTAL							

8 oz

Step 2 – Tracking Food

DINNER	Amount	Cal.	Fat gm	Carb. gm	Fiber gm	Net Carb. gm	Protein gm
TOTAL							

SNACK	Amount	Cal.	Fat gm	Carb. gm	Fiber gm	Net Carb. gm	Protein gm
TOTAL							

| Daily Total | | | | | | | |
| Daily Target | | | | | | | |

Ketone Levels (mM)

0   0.5   1.0   1.5   2.0   2.5   3.0   5.0+

Fasting Clock
Fast start _____
Fast finish _____
Hours fasted _____

Exercise notes
What _____
Duration _____
Calories Burned _____

Vitamins / Supplements / Meds.

Description	Qty

How was today?

_____

_____

DAILY

Date: _____ Mon. Tue. Wed. Thur. Fri. Sat. Sun.

BREAKFAST	Amount	Cal.	Fat gm	Carb. gm	Fiber gm	Net Carb. gm	Protein gm
⊙ TOTAL							

SNACK	Amount	Cal.	Fat gm	Carb. gm	Fiber gm	Net Carb. gm	Protein gm
⊙ TOTAL							

LUNCH	Amount	Cal.	Fat gm	Carb. gm	Fiber gm	Net Carb. gm	Protein gm
⊙ TOTAL							

SNACK	Amount	Cal.	Fat gm	Carb. gm	Fiber gm	Net Carb. gm	Protein gm
⊙ TOTAL							

8 oz

Step 2 – Tracking Food

DINNER	Amount	Cal.	Fat gm	Carb. gm	Fiber gm	Net Carb. gm	Protein gm
TOTAL							

SNACK	Amount	Cal.	Fat gm	Carb. gm	Fiber gm	Net Carb. gm	Protein gm
TOTAL							

| Daily Total | | | | | | | |
| Daily Target | | | | | | | |

Ketone Levels (mM)

0   0.5   1.0   1.5   2.0   2.5   3.0   5.0+

Fasting Clock

Fast start _____   Hours fasted

Fast finish _____

Exercise notes

What _____

Duration _____

Calories Burned _____

Vitamins / Supplements / Meds.

Description	Qty

How was today?

_____

_____

DAILY

Date: _____ Mon. Tue. Wed. Thur. Fri. Sat. Sun.

BREAKFAST	Amount	Cal.	Fat gm	Carb. gm	Fiber gm	Net Carb. gm	Protein gm
TOTAL							

SNACK	Amount	Cal.	Fat gm	Carb. gm	Fiber gm	Net Carb. gm	Protein gm
TOTAL							

LUNCH	Amount	Cal.	Fat gm	Carb. gm	Fiber gm	Net Carb. gm	Protein gm
TOTAL							

SNACK	Amount	Cal.	Fat gm	Carb. gm	Fiber gm	Net Carb. gm	Protein gm
TOTAL							

8 oz

Step 2 – Tracking Food

DINNER	Amount	Cal.	Fat gm	Carb. gm	Fiber gm	Net Carb. gm	Protein gm
TOTAL							

SNACK	Amount	Cal.	Fat gm	Carb. gm	Fiber gm	Net Carb. gm	Protein gm
TOTAL							

| Daily Total | | | | | | | |
| Daily Target | | | | | | | |

Ketone Levels (mM)

0   0.5   1.0   1.5   2.0   2.5   3.0   5.0+

Fasting Clock

Fast start _____   Hours fasted ____

Fast finish _____

Exercise notes

What _____

Duration _____

Calories Burned _____

Vitamins / Supplements / Meds.

Description	Qty

How was today?

_____

_____

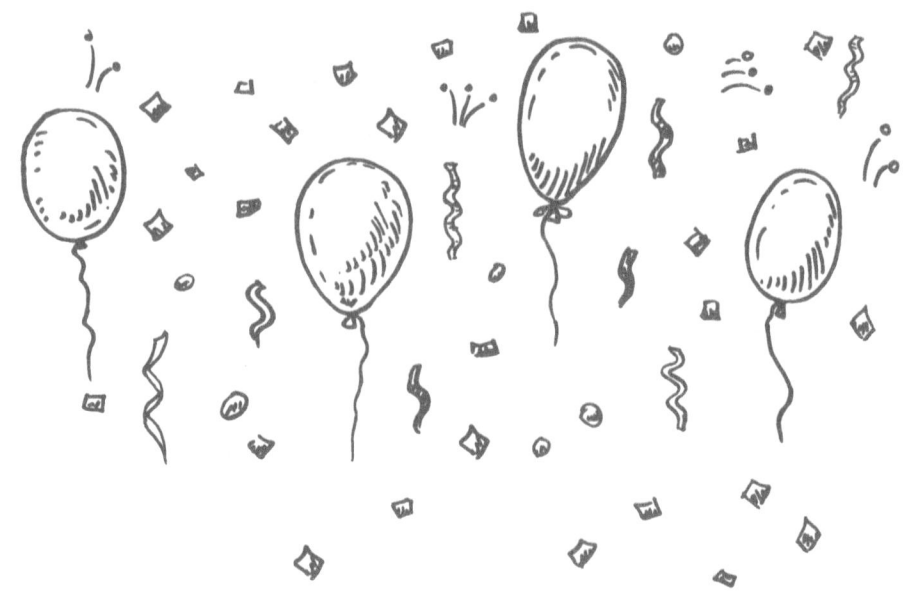

7-DAYS WINNING

Congratulations, you have accomplished 7 days.

Don't forget to celebrate.

WEEKLY REVIEW

This is your first weekly review. It is intended to look back and see how far you have come and make adjustments as you need them for next week.

Checking that you are on the right track to your health goals and learning how to get back if not.

Ideas for the review:

- Is there any blank data which might be useful? Are there any fields which you do not feel are necessary moving forward?

- Are there any patterns emerging? This includes what you are eating, when you are eating it, or how you are feeling?

- Were there any triggers like events, days of the week, or anything else that interrupted you across the week?

There are no right or wrong answers and only you will be looking at this, so be honest.

WEEKLY WINS

What went well this week? What can I take forward to next week?

Making next week even better

What have you learned this week? What could have been better?

I seem to be eating more carbs in the afternoon and evenings, usually snacking on some chips or fruit. There have been some very long meetings at work and there wasn't anything keto in the room.

I am also struggling when out with friends, they always want to go to somewhere that I cannot eat well at.

What can you implement next week to ensure success?

I will buy some keto snacks and take them to work, some nuts or perhaps make some of those yummy fat bombs.

For my friends, I will suggest 'dinner parties' instead. If I propose the first one at my house, I can cook keto and also show them that keto can be delicious.

Do not forget to record any measurements you wish to track weekly in the reference section.

WEEKLY WINS

What went well this week? What can I take forward to next week?

Making next week even better

What have you learned this week? What could have been better?

_____
_____
_____
_____
_____
_____

What can you implement next week to ensure success?

_____
_____
_____
_____
_____

Do not forget to record any measurements you wish to track weekly in the reference section.

WEEK OF ____

Date: Mon.   Tue.   Wed.   Thur.   Fri.   Sat.   Sun.

BREAKFAST	Amount	Cal.	Fat gm	Carb. gm	Fiber gm	Net Carb. gm	Protein gm
TOTAL							

SNACK	Amount	Cal.	Fat gm	Carb. gm	Fiber gm	Net Carb. gm	Protein gm
TOTAL							

LUNCH	Amount	Cal.	Fat gm	Carb. gm	Fiber gm	Net Carb. gm	Protein gm
TOTAL							

SNACK	Amount	Cal.	Fat gm	Carb. gm	Fiber gm	Net Carb. gm	Protein gm
TOTAL							

8 oz

Step 2 – Tracking Food

DINNER	Amount	Cal.	Fat gm	Carb. gm	Fiber gm	Net Carb. gm	Protein gm
TOTAL							

SNACK	Amount	Cal.	Fat gm	Carb. gm	Fiber gm	Net Carb. gm	Protein gm
TOTAL							

| Daily Total | | | | | | | |
| Daily Target | | | | | | | |

Ketone Levels (mM)

0   0.5   1.0   1.5   2.0   2.5   3.0   5.0+

Fasting Clock

Fast start _____

Fast finish _____

Hours fasted

Exercise notes

What _____

Duration _____

Calories Burned _____

Vitamins / Supplements / Meds.

Description	Qty

How was today?

_____

_____

DAILY

Date: _____   Mon. Tue. Wed. Thur. Fri. Sat. Sun.

BREAKFAST	Amount	Cal.	Fat gm	Carb. gm	Fiber gm	Net Carb. gm	Protein gm
🕐 TOTAL							

SNACK	Amount	Cal.	Fat gm	Carb. gm	Fiber gm	Net Carb. gm	Protein gm
🕐 TOTAL							

LUNCH	Amount	Cal.	Fat gm	Carb. gm	Fiber gm	Net Carb. gm	Protein gm
🕐 TOTAL							

SNACK	Amount	Cal.	Fat gm	Carb. gm	Fiber gm	Net Carb. gm	Protein gm
🕐 TOTAL							

8 oz

Step 2 – Tracking Food

DINNER	Amount	Cal.	Fat gm	Carb. gm	Fiber gm	Net Carb. gm	Protein gm
TOTAL							

SNACK	Amount	Cal.	Fat gm	Carb. gm	Fiber gm	Net Carb. gm	Protein gm
TOTAL							

| Daily Total | | | | | | | |
| Daily Target | | | | | | | |

Ketone Levels (mM)

0   0.5   1.0   1.5   2.0   2.5   3.0   5.0+

Fasting Clock

Fast start _____   Hours fasted ____

Fast finish _____

Exercise notes

What _____

Duration _____

Calories Burned _____

Vitamins / Supplements / Meds.

Description	Qty

How was today?

_____

_____

_____

DAILY

Date: Mon.   Tue.   Wed.   Thur.   Fri.   Sat.   Sun.

BREAKFAST	Amount	Cal.	Fat gm	Carb. gm	Fiber gm	Net Carb. gm	Protein gm
⏰ TOTAL							

SNACK	Amount	Cal.	Fat gm	Carb. gm	Fiber gm	Net Carb. gm	Protein gm
⏰ TOTAL							

LUNCH	Amount	Cal.	Fat gm	Carb. gm	Fiber gm	Net Carb. gm	Protein gm
⏰ TOTAL							

SNACK	Amount	Cal.	Fat gm	Carb. gm	Fiber gm	Net Carb. gm	Protein gm
⏰ TOTAL							

8 oz

Step 2 – Tracking Food

DINNER	Amount	Cal.	Fat gm	Carb. gm	Fiber gm	Net Carb. gm	Protein gm
TOTAL							

SNACK	Amount	Cal.	Fat gm	Carb. gm	Fiber gm	Net Carb. gm	Protein gm
TOTAL							
Daily Total							
Daily Target							

Ketone Levels (mM)

0   0.5   1.0   1.5   2.0   2.5   3.0   5.0+

Fasting Clock

Fast start _____

Fast finish _____

Hours fasted

Exercise notes

What _____

Duration _____

Calories Burned_____

Vitamins / Supplements / Meds.

Description	Qty

How was today?

_____

_____

DAILY

Date: Mon. Tue. Wed. Thur. Fri. Sat. Sun.

BREAKFAST	Amount	Cal.	Fat gm	Carb. gm	Fiber gm	Net Carb. gm	Protein gm
TOTAL							

SNACK	Amount	Cal.	Fat gm	Carb. gm	Fiber gm	Net Carb. gm	Protein gm
TOTAL							

LUNCH	Amount	Cal.	Fat gm	Carb. gm	Fiber gm	Net Carb. gm	Protein gm
TOTAL							

SNACK	Amount	Cal.	Fat gm	Carb. gm	Fiber gm	Net Carb. gm	Protein gm
TOTAL							

8 oz

Step 2 – Tracking Food

DINNER	Amount	Cal.	Fat gm	Carb. gm	Fiber gm	Net Carb. gm	Protein gm
TOTAL							

SNACK	Amount	Cal.	Fat gm	Carb. gm	Fiber gm	Net Carb. gm	Protein gm
TOTAL							

| Daily Total | | | | | | | |
| Daily Target | | | | | | | |

Ketone Levels (mM)
0   0.5   1.0   1.5   2.0   2.5   3.0   5.0+

Fasting Clock
Fast start _____
Fast finish _____
Hours fasted _____

Exercise notes
What _____
Duration _____
Calories Burned _____

Vitamins / Supplements / Meds.

Description	Qty

How was today?
_____
_____

DAILY

Date: _____   Mon. Tue. Wed. Thur. Fri. Sat. Sun.

BREAKFAST	Amount	Cal.	Fat gm	Carb. gm	Fiber gm	Net Carb. gm	Protein gm
⊙ TOTAL							

SNACK	Amount	Cal.	Fat gm	Carb. gm	Fiber gm	Net Carb. gm	Protein gm
⊙ TOTAL							

LUNCH	Amount	Cal.	Fat gm	Carb. gm	Fiber gm	Net Carb. gm	Protein gm
⊙ TOTAL							

SNACK	Amount	Cal.	Fat gm	Carb. gm	Fiber gm	Net Carb. gm	Protein gm
⊙ TOTAL							

8 oz

Step 2 – Tracking Food

DINNER	Amount	Cal.	Fat gm	Carb. gm	Fiber gm	Net Carb. gm	Protein gm
TOTAL							

SNACK	Amount	Cal.	Fat gm	Carb. gm	Fiber gm	Net Carb. gm	Protein gm
TOTAL							
Daily Total							
Daily Target							

Ketone Levels (mM)

0   0.5   1.0   1.5   2.0   2.5   3.0   5.0+

Fasting Clock
Fast start _____
Fast finish _____
Hours fasted

Exercise notes
What _____
Duration _____
Calories Burned _____

Vitamins / Supplements / Meds.

Description	Qty

How was today?

_____
_____

DAILY

Date: _____ Mon. Tue. Wed. Thur. Fri. Sat. Sun.

BREAKFAST	Amount	Cal.	Fat gm	Carb. gm	Fiber gm	Net Carb. gm	Protein gm
🕐 TOTAL							

SNACK	Amount	Cal.	Fat gm	Carb. gm	Fiber gm	Net Carb. gm	Protein gm
🕐 TOTAL							

LUNCH	Amount	Cal.	Fat gm	Carb. gm	Fiber gm	Net Carb. gm	Protein gm
🕐 TOTAL							

SNACK	Amount	Cal.	Fat gm	Carb. gm	Fiber gm	Net Carb. gm	Protein gm
🕐 TOTAL							

8 oz

Step 2 – Tracking Food

DINNER	Amount	Cal.	Fat gm	Carb. gm	Fiber gm	Net Carb. gm	Protein gm
🕐 TOTAL							

SNACK	Amount	Cal.	Fat gm	Carb. gm	Fiber gm	Net Carb. gm	Protein gm
🕐 TOTAL							

| Daily Total | | | | | | | |
| Daily Target | | | | | | | |

Ketone Levels (mM)

|—|—|—|—|—|—|—|
0   0.5   1.0   1.5   2.0   2.5   3.0   5.0+

Fasting Clock

Fast start _____   Hours fasted

Fast finish _____

Exercise notes

What _____

Duration _____

Calories Burned _____

Vitamins / Supplements / Meds.

Description	Qty

How was today?

_____

_____

DAILY

Date: _____ Mon. Tue. Wed. Thur. Fri. Sat. Sun.

BREAKFAST	Amount	Cal.	Fat gm	Carb. gm	Fiber gm	Net Carb. gm	Protein gm
TOTAL							

SNACK	Amount	Cal.	Fat gm	Carb. gm	Fiber gm	Net Carb. gm	Protein gm
TOTAL							

LUNCH	Amount	Cal.	Fat gm	Carb. gm	Fiber gm	Net Carb. gm	Protein gm
TOTAL							

SNACK	Amount	Cal.	Fat gm	Carb. gm	Fiber gm	Net Carb. gm	Protein gm
TOTAL							

8 oz

Step 2 – Tracking Food

DINNER	Amount	Cal.	Fat gm	Carb. gm	Fiber gm	Net Carb. gm	Protein gm
🕒 TOTAL							

SNACK	Amount	Cal.	Fat gm	Carb. gm	Fiber gm	Net Carb. gm	Protein gm
🕒 TOTAL							

| Daily Total | | | | | | | |
| Daily Target | | | | | | | |

Ketone Levels (mM)

|—|—|—|—|—|—|—|
0   0.5   1.0   1.5   2.0   2.5   3.0   5.0+

Fasting Clock

Fast start _____   Hours fasted

Fast finish _____

Exercise notes

What _____

Duration _____

Calories Burned _____

Vitamins / Supplements / Meds.

Description	Qty

How was today?

_____

_____

WEEKLY WINS

What went well this week? What can I take forward to next week?

Making next week even better

What have you learned this week? What could have been better?

_____

_____

_____

_____

_____

_____

What can you implement next week to ensure success?

_____

_____

_____

_____

_____

_____

Do not forget to record any measurements you wish to track weekly in the reference section.

> **"THE BODY IS LIKE A PIANO, AND HAPPINESS IS LIKE MUSIC. IT IS NEEDFUL TO HAVE THE INSTRUMENT IN GOOD ORDER"**

WEEK OF ____

Date: _____   Mon. Tue. Wed. Thur. Fri. Sat. Sun.

BREAKFAST	Amount	Cal.	Fat gm	Carb. gm	Fiber gm	Net Carb. gm	Protein gm
🕒 TOTAL							

SNACK	Amount	Cal.	Fat gm	Carb. gm	Fiber gm	Net Carb. gm	Protein gm
🕒 TOTAL							

LUNCH	Amount	Cal.	Fat gm	Carb. gm	Fiber gm	Net Carb. gm	Protein gm
🕒 TOTAL							

SNACK	Amount	Cal.	Fat gm	Carb. gm	Fiber gm	Net Carb. gm	Protein gm
🕒 TOTAL							

        8 oz

Step 2 – Tracking Food

DINNER	Amount	Cal.	Fat gm	Carb. gm	Fiber gm	Net Carb. gm	Protein gm
🕐 TOTAL							

SNACK	Amount	Cal.	Fat gm	Carb. gm	Fiber gm	Net Carb. gm	Protein gm
🕐 TOTAL							

| Daily Total | | | | | | | |
| Daily Target | | | | | | | |

Ketone Levels (mM)

|—+—+—+—+—+—+—|
0   0.5   1.0   1.5   2.0   2.5   3.0   5.0+

Fasting Clock

Fast start _____

Fast finish _____

Hours fasted [ ]

Exercise notes

What _____

Duration _____

Calories Burned _____

Vitamins / Supplements / Meds.

Description	Qty

How was today?

_____

_____

DAILY

Date: Mon. Tue. Wed. Thur. Fri. Sat. Sun.

BREAKFAST	Amount	Cal.	Fat gm	Carb. gm	Fiber gm	Net Carb. gm	Protein gm
TOTAL							

SNACK	Amount	Cal.	Fat gm	Carb. gm	Fiber gm	Net Carb. gm	Protein gm
TOTAL							

LUNCH	Amount	Cal.	Fat gm	Carb. gm	Fiber gm	Net Carb. gm	Protein gm
TOTAL							

SNACK	Amount	Cal.	Fat gm	Carb. gm	Fiber gm	Net Carb. gm	Protein gm
TOTAL							

8 oz

Step 2 – Tracking Food

DINNER	Amount	Cal.	Fat gm	Carb. gm	Fiber gm	Net Carb. gm	Protein gm
🕐 TOTAL							

SNACK	Amount	Cal.	Fat gm	Carb. gm	Fiber gm	Net Carb. gm	Protein gm
🕐 TOTAL							

| Daily Total | | | | | | | |
| Daily Target | | | | | | | |

Ketone Levels (mM)

0   0.5   1.0   1.5   2.0   2.5   3.0   5.0+

Fasting Clock

Fast start _____   Hours fasted

Fast finish _____

Exercise notes

What _____

Duration _____

Calories Burned _____

Vitamins / Supplements / Meds.

Description	Qty

How was today?

_____

_____

DAILY

Date: _____   Mon. Tue. Wed. Thur. Fri. Sat. Sun.

BREAKFAST	Amount	Cal.	Fat gm	Carb. gm	Fiber gm	Net Carb. gm	Protein gm
⊙ TOTAL							

SNACK	Amount	Cal.	Fat gm	Carb. gm	Fiber gm	Net Carb. gm	Protein gm
⊙ TOTAL							

LUNCH	Amount	Cal.	Fat gm	Carb. gm	Fiber gm	Net Carb. gm	Protein gm
⊙ TOTAL							

SNACK	Amount	Cal.	Fat gm	Carb. gm	Fiber gm	Net Carb. gm	Protein gm
⊙ TOTAL							

8 oz

Step 2 – Tracking Food

DINNER	Amount	Cal.	Fat gm	Carb. gm	Fiber gm	Net Carb. gm	Protein gm
TOTAL							

SNACK	Amount	Cal.	Fat gm	Carb. gm	Fiber gm	Net Carb. gm	Protein gm
TOTAL							

Daily Total							
Daily Target							

Ketone Levels (mM)

0   0.5   1.0   1.5   2.0   2.5   3.0   5.0+

Fasting Clock

Fast start _____   Hours fasted ____

Fast finish _____

Exercise notes

What _____

Duration _____

Calories Burned _____

Vitamins / Supplements / Meds.

Description	Qty

How was today?

_____

_____

DAILY

Date: _____   Mon. Tue. Wed. Thur. Fri. Sat. Sun.

BREAKFAST	Amount	Cal.	Fat gm	Carb. gm	Fiber gm	Net Carb. gm	Protein gm
🕐 TOTAL							

SNACK	Amount	Cal.	Fat gm	Carb. gm	Fiber gm	Net Carb. gm	Protein gm
🕐 TOTAL							

LUNCH	Amount	Cal.	Fat gm	Carb. gm	Fiber gm	Net Carb. gm	Protein gm
🕐 TOTAL							

SNACK	Amount	Cal.	Fat gm	Carb. gm	Fiber gm	Net Carb. gm	Protein gm
🕐 TOTAL							

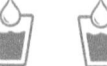 8 oz

Step 2 – Tracking Food

DINNER	Amount	Cal.	Fat gm	Carb. gm	Fiber gm	Net Carb. gm	Protein gm
TOTAL							

SNACK	Amount	Cal.	Fat gm	Carb. gm	Fiber gm	Net Carb. gm	Protein gm
TOTAL							

| Daily Total | | | | | | | |
| Daily Target | | | | | | | |

Ketone Levels (mM)

0   0.5   1.0   1.5   2.0   2.5   3.0   5.0+

Fasting Clock

Fast start _____   Hours fasted

Fast finish _____

Exercise notes

What _____

Duration _____

Calories Burned _____

Vitamins / Supplements / Meds.

Description	Qty

How was today?

_____

_____

DAILY

Date: Mon.   Tue.   Wed.   Thur.   Fri.   Sat.   Sun.

BREAKFAST	Amount	Cal.	Fat gm	Carb. gm	Fiber gm	Net Carb. gm	Protein gm
⏱ TOTAL							

SNACK	Amount	Cal.	Fat gm	Carb. gm	Fiber gm	Net Carb. gm	Protein gm
⏱ TOTAL							

LUNCH	Amount	Cal.	Fat gm	Carb. gm	Fiber gm	Net Carb. gm	Protein gm
⏱ TOTAL							

SNACK	Amount	Cal.	Fat gm	Carb. gm	Fiber gm	Net Carb. gm	Protein gm
⏱ TOTAL							

    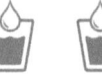

8 oz

Step 2 – Tracking Food

DINNER	Amount	Cal.	Fat gm	Carb. gm	Fiber gm	Net Carb. gm	Protein gm
⏰ TOTAL							

SNACK	Amount	Cal.	Fat gm	Carb. gm	Fiber gm	Net Carb. gm	Protein gm
⏰ TOTAL							

| Daily Total | | | | | | | |
| Daily Target | | | | | | | |

Ketone Levels (mM)

| — | — | — | — | — | — | — |
| 0 | 0.5 | 1.0 | 1.5 | 2.0 | 2.5 | 3.0 | 5.0+ |

Fasting Clock

Fast start _____

Fast finish _____

Hours fasted

Exercise notes

What _____

Duration _____

Calories Burned _____

Vitamins / Supplements / Meds.

Description	Qty

How was today?

_____

_____

DAILY

Date: _____   Mon.   Tue.   Wed.   Thur.   Fri.   Sat.   Sun.

BREAKFAST	Amount	Cal.	Fat gm	Carb. gm	Fiber gm	Net Carb. gm	Protein gm
🕒 TOTAL							

SNACK	Amount	Cal.	Fat gm	Carb. gm	Fiber gm	Net Carb. gm	Protein gm
🕒 TOTAL							

LUNCH	Amount	Cal.	Fat gm	Carb. gm	Fiber gm	Net Carb. gm	Protein gm
🕒 TOTAL							

SNACK	Amount	Cal.	Fat gm	Carb. gm	Fiber gm	Net Carb. gm	Protein gm
🕒 TOTAL							

🥛 🥛 🥛 🥛 🥛 🥛 🥛 🥛   8 oz

Step 2 – Tracking Food

DINNER	Amount	Cal.	Fat gm	Carb. gm	Fiber gm	Net Carb. gm	Protein gm
TOTAL							

SNACK	Amount	Cal.	Fat gm	Carb. gm	Fiber gm	Net Carb. gm	Protein gm
TOTAL							

| Daily Total | | | | | | | |
| Daily Target | | | | | | | |

Ketone Levels (mM)

| 0 | 0.5 | 1.0 | 1.5 | 2.0 | 2.5 | 3.0 | 5.0+ |

Fasting Clock

Fast start _____

Fast finish _____

Hours fasted ☐

Exercise notes

What _____

Duration _____

Calories Burned _____

Vitamins / Supplements / Meds.

Description	Qty

How was today?

_____

_____

DAILY

Date: _____   Mon. Tue. Wed. Thur. Fri. Sat. Sun.

BREAKFAST	Amount	Cal.	Fat gm	Carb. gm	Fiber gm	Net Carb. gm	Protein gm
🕐 TOTAL							

SNACK	Amount	Cal.	Fat gm	Carb. gm	Fiber gm	Net Carb. gm	Protein gm
🕐 TOTAL							

LUNCH	Amount	Cal.	Fat gm	Carb. gm	Fiber gm	Net Carb. gm	Protein gm
🕐 TOTAL							

SNACK	Amount	Cal.	Fat gm	Carb. gm	Fiber gm	Net Carb. gm	Protein gm
🕐 TOTAL							

8 oz

Step 2 – Tracking Food

DINNER	Amount	Cal.	Fat gm	Carb. gm	Fiber gm	Net Carb. gm	Protein gm
TOTAL							

SNACK	Amount	Cal.	Fat gm	Carb. gm	Fiber gm	Net Carb. gm	Protein gm
TOTAL							
Daily Total							
Daily Target							

Ketone Levels (mM)

|—|—|—|—|—|—|—|
0   0.5   1.0   1.5   2.0   2.5   3.0   5.0+

Fasting Clock

Fast start _____   Hours fasted

Fast finish _____

Exercise notes

What _____

Duration _____

Calories Burned _____

Vitamins / Supplements / Meds.

Description	Qty

How was today?

_____

_____

_____

WEEKLY WINS

What went well this week? What can I take forward to next week?

Making next week even better

What have you learned this week? What could have been better?

_____

_____

_____

_____

_____

_____

What can you implement next week to ensure success?

_____

_____

_____

_____

_____

_____

Do not forget to record any measurements you wish to track weekly in the reference section.

> **"IF YOU KEEP GOOD FOOD IN YOUR FRIDGE, YOU WILL EAT GOODFOOD"**

WEEK OF ____

Date: _____ Mon. Tue. Wed. Thur. Fri. Sat. Sun.

BREAKFAST	Amount	Cal.	Fat gm	Carb. gm	Fiber gm	Net Carb. gm	Protein gm
🕐 TOTAL							

SNACK	Amount	Cal.	Fat gm	Carb. gm	Fiber gm	Net Carb. gm	Protein gm
🕐 TOTAL							

LUNCH	Amount	Cal.	Fat gm	Carb. gm	Fiber gm	Net Carb. gm	Protein gm
🕐 TOTAL							

SNACK	Amount	Cal.	Fat gm	Carb. gm	Fiber gm	Net Carb. gm	Protein gm
🕐 TOTAL							

8 oz

Step 2 – Tracking Food

DINNER	Amount	Cal.	Fat gm	Carb. gm	Fiber gm	Net Carb. gm	Protein gm
🕒 TOTAL							

SNACK	Amount	Cal.	Fat gm	Carb. gm	Fiber gm	Net Carb. gm	Protein gm
🕒 TOTAL							
Daily Total							
Daily Target							

Ketone Levels (mM)

|—|—|—|—|—|—|—|
0   0.5 1.0 1.5 2.0 2.5 3.0   5.0+

Fasting Clock

Fast start _____   Hours fasted [ ]

Fast finish _____

Exercise notes

What _____

Duration _____

Calories Burned _____

Vitamins / Supplements / Meds.

Description	Qty

How was today?

_____

_____

DAILY

Date: _____   Mon. Tue. Wed. Thur. Fri. Sat. Sun.

BREAKFAST	Amount	Cal.	Fat gm	Carb. gm	Fiber gm	Net Carb. gm	Protein gm
🕐 TOTAL							

SNACK	Amount	Cal.	Fat gm	Carb. gm	Fiber gm	Net Carb. gm	Protein gm
🕐 TOTAL							

LUNCH	Amount	Cal.	Fat gm	Carb. gm	Fiber gm	Net Carb. gm	Protein gm
🕐 TOTAL							

SNACK	Amount	Cal.	Fat gm	Carb. gm	Fiber gm	Net Carb. gm	Protein gm
🕐 TOTAL							

▽ ▽ ▽ ▽ ▽ ▽ ▽ ▽ 8 oz

Step 2 – Tracking Food

DINNER	Amount	Cal.	Fat gm	Carb. gm	Fiber gm	Net Carb. gm	Protein gm
TOTAL							

SNACK	Amount	Cal.	Fat gm	Carb. gm	Fiber gm	Net Carb. gm	Protein gm
TOTAL							

Daily Total						
Daily Target						

Ketone Levels (mM)

0   0.5   1.0   1.5   2.0   2.5   3.0   5.0+

Fasting Clock

Fast start _____   Hours fasted

Fast finish _____

Exercise notes

What _____

Duration _____

Calories Burned _____

Vitamins / Supplements / Meds.

Description	Qty

How was today?

_____

_____

_____

DAILY

Date: _____ Mon. Tue. Wed. Thur. Fri. Sat. Sun.

BREAKFAST	Amount	Cal.	Fat gm	Carb. gm	Fiber gm	Net Carb. gm	Protein gm
🕐 TOTAL							

SNACK	Amount	Cal.	Fat gm	Carb. gm	Fiber gm	Net Carb. gm	Protein gm
🕐 TOTAL							

LUNCH	Amount	Cal.	Fat gm	Carb. gm	Fiber gm	Net Carb. gm	Protein gm
🕐 TOTAL							

SNACK	Amount	Cal.	Fat gm	Carb. gm	Fiber gm	Net Carb. gm	Protein gm
🕐 TOTAL							

🥛 🥛 🥛 🥛 🥛 🥛 🥛 🥛   8 oz

Step 2 – Tracking Food

DINNER	Amount	Cal.	Fat gm	Carb. gm	Fiber gm	Net Carb. gm	Protein gm
TOTAL							

SNACK	Amount	Cal.	Fat gm	Carb. gm	Fiber gm	Net Carb. gm	Protein gm
TOTAL							

Daily Total	
Daily Target	

Ketone Levels (mM)

|—|—|—|—|—|—|—|
0   0.5 1.0 1.5 2.0 2.5 3.0   5.0+

Fasting Clock
Fast start _____   Hours fasted
Fast finish _____   [   ]

Exercise notes
What _____
Duration _____
Calories Burned _____

Vitamins / Supplements / Meds.

Description	Qty

How was today?
_____
_____

DAILY

Date: _____ Mon. Tue. Wed. Thur. Fri. Sat. Sun.

BREAKFAST	Amount	Cal.	Fat gm	Carb. gm	Fiber gm	Net Carb. gm	Protein gm
ⓞ TOTAL							

SNACK	Amount	Cal.	Fat gm	Carb. gm	Fiber gm	Net Carb. gm	Protein gm
ⓞ TOTAL							

LUNCH	Amount	Cal.	Fat gm	Carb. gm	Fiber gm	Net Carb. gm	Protein gm
ⓞ TOTAL							

SNACK	Amount	Cal.	Fat gm	Carb. gm	Fiber gm	Net Carb. gm	Protein gm
ⓞ TOTAL							

8 oz

Step 2 – Tracking Food

DINNER	Amount	Cal.	Fat gm	Carb. gm	Fiber gm	Net Carb. gm	Protein gm
TOTAL							

SNACK	Amount	Cal.	Fat gm	Carb. gm	Fiber gm	Net Carb. gm	Protein gm
TOTAL							

| Daily Total | | | | | | | |
| Daily Target | | | | | | | |

Ketone Levels (mM)

0   0.5   1.0   1.5   2.0   2.5   3.0   5.0+

Fasting Clock

Fast start _____

Fast finish _____

Hours fasted _____

Exercise notes

What _____

Duration _____

Calories Burned _____

Vitamins / Supplements / Meds.

Description	Qty

How was today?

_____

_____

DAILY

Date: _____ Mon. Tue. Wed. Thur. Fri. Sat. Sun.

BREAKFAST	Amount	Cal.	Fat gm	Carb. gm	Fiber gm	Net Carb. gm	Protein gm
TOTAL							

SNACK	Amount	Cal.	Fat gm	Carb. gm	Fiber gm	Net Carb. gm	Protein gm
TOTAL							

LUNCH	Amount	Cal.	Fat gm	Carb. gm	Fiber gm	Net Carb. gm	Protein gm
TOTAL							

SNACK	Amount	Cal.	Fat gm	Carb. gm	Fiber gm	Net Carb. gm	Protein gm
TOTAL							

8 oz

Step 2 – Tracking Food

DINNER	Amount	Cal.	Fat gm	Carb. gm	Fiber gm	Net Carb. gm	Protein gm
⏱ TOTAL							

SNACK	Amount	Cal.	Fat gm	Carb. gm	Fiber gm	Net Carb. gm	Protein gm
⏱ TOTAL							
Daily Total							
Daily Target							

Ketone Levels (mM)

| 0 | 0.5 | 1.0 | 1.5 | 2.0 | 2.5 | 3.0 | 5.0+ |

Fasting Clock

Fast start _____

Fast finish _____

Hours fasted _____

Exercise notes

What _____

Duration _____

Calories Burned _____

Vitamins / Supplements / Meds.

Description	Qty

How was today?

_____

_____

DAILY

Date: _____   Mon. Tue. Wed. Thur. Fri. Sat. Sun.

BREAKFAST	Amount	Cal.	Fat gm	Carb. gm	Fiber gm	Net Carb. gm	Protein gm
⊙ TOTAL							

SNACK	Amount	Cal.	Fat gm	Carb. gm	Fiber gm	Net Carb. gm	Protein gm
⊙ TOTAL							

LUNCH	Amount	Cal.	Fat gm	Carb. gm	Fiber gm	Net Carb. gm	Protein gm
⊙ TOTAL							

SNACK	Amount	Cal.	Fat gm	Carb. gm	Fiber gm	Net Carb. gm	Protein gm
⊙ TOTAL							

8 oz

Step 2 – Tracking Food

DINNER	Amount	Cal.	Fat gm	Carb. gm	Fiber gm	Net Carb. gm	Protein gm
TOTAL							

SNACK	Amount	Cal.	Fat gm	Carb. gm	Fiber gm	Net Carb. gm	Protein gm
TOTAL							

| Daily Total | | | | | | | |
| Daily Target | | | | | | | |

Ketone Levels (mM)

0   0.5   1.0   1.5   2.0   2.5   3.0   5.0+

Fasting Clock

Fast start _____

Fast finish _____

Hours fasted _____

Exercise notes

What _____

Duration _____

Calories Burned _____

Vitamins / Supplements / Meds.

Description	Qty

How was today?

_____

_____

DAILY

Date: _____ Mon. Tue. Wed. Thur. Fri. Sat. Sun.

BREAKFAST	Amount	Cal.	Fat gm	Carb. gm	Fiber gm	Net Carb. gm	Protein gm
⊘ TOTAL							

SNACK	Amount	Cal.	Fat gm	Carb. gm	Fiber gm	Net Carb. gm	Protein gm
⊘ TOTAL							

LUNCH	Amount	Cal.	Fat gm	Carb. gm	Fiber gm	Net Carb. gm	Protein gm
⊘ TOTAL							

SNACK	Amount	Cal.	Fat gm	Carb. gm	Fiber gm	Net Carb. gm	Protein gm
⊘ TOTAL							

 8 oz

Step 2 – Tracking Food

DINNER	Amount	Cal.	Fat gm	Carb. gm	Fiber gm	Net Carb. gm	Protein gm
TOTAL							

SNACK	Amount	Cal.	Fat gm	Carb. gm	Fiber gm	Net Carb. gm	Protein gm
TOTAL							
Daily Total							
Daily Target							

Ketone Levels (mM)

0   0.5   1.0   1.5   2.0   2.5   3.0   5.0+

Fasting Clock
Fast start _____   Hours fasted
Fast finish _____

Exercise notes
What _____
Duration _____
Calories Burned _____

Vitamins / Supplements / Meds.

Description	Qty

How was today?

_____
_____
_____

28-DAYS WINNING

Congratulations, you have now completed an entire month of journaling and you should be seeing some very positive results from your hard work.

Take this time to reflect on your progress and how far you have come. Look back at your charts and the changes you've made. Be proud and recommit to another 28 days.

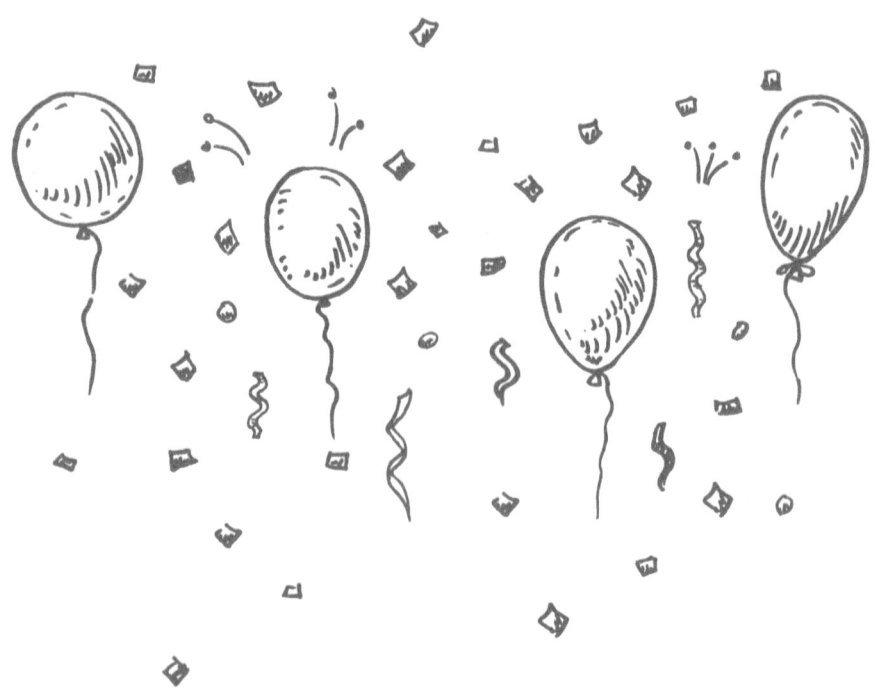

WEEKLY REVIEW

This is your first weekly review. It is intended to look back and see how far you have come and make adjustments as you need them for next week.

Checking that you are on the right track to your health goals and learning how to get back if not.

Ideas for the review:

- Is there any blank data which might be useful? Are there any fields which you do not feel are necessary moving forward?

- Are there any patterns emerging? This includes what you are eating, when you are eating it, or how you are feeling?

- Were there any triggers like events, days of the week, or anything else that interrupted you across during the week?

There are no right or wrong answers and only you will be looking at this, so be honest.

WEEKLY WINS

What went well this week? What can I take forward to next week?

Making next week even better

What have you learned this week? What could have been better?

_____

_____

_____

_____

_____

_____

What can you implement next week to ensure success?

_____

_____

_____

_____

_____

_____

Do not forget to record any measurements you wish to track weekly in the reference section.

"FALL IN LOVE WITH THE PROCESS AND THE RESULTS WILL COME"

WEEK OF ____

Date: Mon.   Tue.   Wed.   Thur.   Fri.   Sat.   Sun.

BREAKFAST	Amount	Cal.	Fat gm	Carb. gm	Fiber gm	Net Carb. gm	Protein gm
🕐 TOTAL							

SNACK	Amount	Cal.	Fat gm	Carb. gm	Fiber gm	Net Carb. gm	Protein gm
🕐 TOTAL							

LUNCH	Amount	Cal.	Fat gm	Carb. gm	Fiber gm	Net Carb. gm	Protein gm
🕐 TOTAL							

SNACK	Amount	Cal.	Fat gm	Carb. gm	Fiber gm	Net Carb. gm	Protein gm
🕐 TOTAL							

8 oz

Step 2 – Tracking Food

DINNER	Amount	Cal.	Fat gm	Carb. gm	Fiber gm	Net Carb. gm	Protein gm
🕐 TOTAL							

SNACK	Amount	Cal.	Fat gm	Carb. gm	Fiber gm	Net Carb. gm	Protein gm
🕐 TOTAL							

| Daily Total | | | | | | | |
| Daily Target | | | | | | | |

Ketone Levels (mM)

|—|—|—|—|—|—|—|
0   0.5   1.0   1.5   2.0   2.5   3.0   5.0+

Fasting Clock

Fast start _____   Hours fasted

Fast finish _____

Exercise notes

What _____

Duration _____

Calories Burned _____

Vitamins / Supplements / Meds.

Description	Qty

How was today?

_____

_____

DAILY

Date: _____   Mon. Tue. Wed. Thur. Fri. Sat. Sun.

BREAKFAST	Amount	Cal.	Fat gm	Carb. gm	Fiber gm	Net Carb. gm	Protein gm
🕐 TOTAL							

SNACK	Amount	Cal.	Fat gm	Carb. gm	Fiber gm	Net Carb. gm	Protein gm
🕐 TOTAL							

LUNCH	Amount	Cal.	Fat gm	Carb. gm	Fiber gm	Net Carb. gm	Protein gm
🕐 TOTAL							

SNACK	Amount	Cal.	Fat gm	Carb. gm	Fiber gm	Net Carb. gm	Protein gm
🕐 TOTAL							

8 oz

Step 2 – Tracking Food

DINNER	Amount	Cal.	Fat gm	Carb. gm	Fiber gm	Net Carb. gm	Protein gm
TOTAL							

SNACK	Amount	Cal.	Fat gm	Carb. gm	Fiber gm	Net Carb. gm	Protein gm
TOTAL							

| Daily Total | | | | | | | |
| Daily Target | | | | | | | |

Ketone Levels (mM)

0   0.5   1.0   1.5   2.0   2.5   3.0   5.0+

Fasting Clock

Fast start _____   Hours fasted [   ]

Fast finish _____

Exercise notes

What _____

Duration _____

Calories Burned _____

Vitamins / Supplements / Meds.

Description	Qty

How was today?

_____

_____

DAILY

Date: Mon. Tue. Wed. Thur. Fri. Sat. Sun.

BREAKFAST	Amount	Cal.	Fat gm	Carb. gm	Fiber gm	Net Carb. gm	Protein gm
🕐 TOTAL							

SNACK	Amount	Cal.	Fat gm	Carb. gm	Fiber gm	Net Carb. gm	Protein gm
🕐 TOTAL							

LUNCH	Amount	Cal.	Fat gm	Carb. gm	Fiber gm	Net Carb. gm	Protein gm
🕐 TOTAL							

SNACK	Amount	Cal.	Fat gm	Carb. gm	Fiber gm	Net Carb. gm	Protein gm
🕐 TOTAL							

8 oz

Step 2 – Tracking Food

DINNER	Amount	Cal.	Fat gm	Carb. gm	Fiber gm	Net Carb. gm	Protein gm
⏲ TOTAL							

SNACK	Amount	Cal.	Fat gm	Carb. gm	Fiber gm	Net Carb. gm	Protein gm
⏲ TOTAL							
Daily Total							
Daily Target							

Ketone Levels (mM)

|—|—|—|—|—|—|—|
0   0.5   1.0   1.5   2.0   2.5   3.0   5.0+

Fasting Clock

Fast start _____   Hours fasted

Fast finish _____

Exercise notes

What _____

Duration _____

Calories Burned _____

Vitamins / Supplements / Meds.

Description	Qty

How was today?

_____

_____

DAILY

Date: _____ Mon. Tue. Wed. Thur. Fri. Sat. Sun.

BREAKFAST	Amount	Cal.	Fat gm	Carb. gm	Fiber gm	Net Carb. gm	Protein gm
🕒 TOTAL							

SNACK	Amount	Cal.	Fat gm	Carb. gm	Fiber gm	Net Carb. gm	Protein gm
🕒 TOTAL							

LUNCH	Amount	Cal.	Fat gm	Carb. gm	Fiber gm	Net Carb. gm	Protein gm
🕒 TOTAL							

SNACK	Amount	Cal.	Fat gm	Carb. gm	Fiber gm	Net Carb. gm	Protein gm
🕒 TOTAL							

8 oz

Step 2 – Tracking Food

DINNER	Amount	Cal.	Fat gm	Carb. gm	Fiber gm	Net Carb. gm	Protein gm
🕐 TOTAL							

SNACK	Amount	Cal.	Fat gm	Carb. gm	Fiber gm	Net Carb. gm	Protein gm
🕐 TOTAL							

| Daily Total | | | | | | | |
| Daily Target | | | | | | | |

Ketone Levels (mM)

|—|—|—|—|—|—|—|
0   0.5   1.0   1.5   2.0   2.5   3.0   5.0+

Fasting Clock

Fast start _____   Hours fasted [   ]

Fast finish _____

Exercise notes

What _____

Duration _____

Calories Burned _____

Vitamins / Supplements / Meds.

Description	Qty

How was today?

_____

_____

DAILY

Date: _____ Mon. Tue. Wed. Thur. Fri. Sat. Sun.

BREAKFAST	Amount	Cal.	Fat gm	Carb. gm	Fiber gm	Net Carb. gm	Protein gm
🕐 TOTAL							

SNACK	Amount	Cal.	Fat gm	Carb. gm	Fiber gm	Net Carb. gm	Protein gm
🕐 TOTAL							

LUNCH	Amount	Cal.	Fat gm	Carb. gm	Fiber gm	Net Carb. gm	Protein gm
🕐 TOTAL							

SNACK	Amount	Cal.	Fat gm	Carb. gm	Fiber gm	Net Carb. gm	Protein gm
🕐 TOTAL							

        8 oz

Step 2 – Tracking Food

DINNER	Amount	Cal.	Fat gm	Carb. gm	Fiber gm	Net Carb. gm	Protein gm
TOTAL							

SNACK	Amount	Cal.	Fat gm	Carb. gm	Fiber gm	Net Carb. gm	Protein gm
TOTAL							

| Daily Total | | | | | | | |
| Daily Target | | | | | | | |

Ketone Levels (mM)

0   0.5   1.0   1.5   2.0   2.5   3.0   5.0+

Fasting Clock

Fast start _____   Hours fasted _____

Fast finish _____

Exercise notes

What _____

Duration _____

Calories Burned _____

Vitamins / Supplements / Meds.

Description	Qty

How was today?

_____

_____

DAILY

Date: _____   Mon. Tue. Wed. Thur. Fri. Sat. Sun.

BREAKFAST	Amount	Cal.	Fat gm	Carb. gm	Fiber gm	Net Carb. gm	Protein gm
🕐 TOTAL							

SNACK	Amount	Cal.	Fat gm	Carb. gm	Fiber gm	Net Carb. gm	Protein gm
🕐 TOTAL							

LUNCH	Amount	Cal.	Fat gm	Carb. gm	Fiber gm	Net Carb. gm	Protein gm
🕐 TOTAL							

SNACK	Amount	Cal.	Fat gm	Carb. gm	Fiber gm	Net Carb. gm	Protein gm
🕐 TOTAL							

8 oz

Step 2 – Tracking Food

DINNER	Amount	Cal.	Fat gm	Carb. gm	Fiber gm	Net Carb. gm	Protein gm
⊙ TOTAL							

SNACK	Amount	Cal.	Fat gm	Carb. gm	Fiber gm	Net Carb. gm	Protein gm
⊙ TOTAL							

| Daily Total | | | | | | | |
| Daily Target | | | | | | | |

Ketone Levels (mM)

├──┼──┼──┼──┼──┼──┤
0   0.5   1.0   1.5   2.0   2.5   3.0   5.0+

Fasting Clock

Fast start _____   Hours fasted

Fast finish _____

Exercise notes

What _____

Duration _____

Calories Burned _____

Vitamins / Supplements / Meds.

Description	Qty

How was today?

_____

_____

DAILY

Date: _____ Mon. Tue. Wed. Thur. Fri. Sat. Sun.

BREAKFAST	Amount	Cal.	Fat gm	Carb. gm	Fiber gm	Net Carb. gm	Protein gm
🕐 TOTAL							

SNACK	Amount	Cal.	Fat gm	Carb. gm	Fiber gm	Net Carb. gm	Protein gm
🕐 TOTAL							

LUNCH	Amount	Cal.	Fat gm	Carb. gm	Fiber gm	Net Carb. gm	Protein gm
🕐 TOTAL							

SNACK	Amount	Cal.	Fat gm	Carb. gm	Fiber gm	Net Carb. gm	Protein gm
🕐 TOTAL							

8 oz

Step 2 – Tracking Food

DINNER	Amount	Cal.	Fat gm	Carb. gm	Fiber gm	Net Carb. gm	Protein gm
🕒 TOTAL							

SNACK	Amount	Cal.	Fat gm	Carb. gm	Fiber gm	Net Carb. gm	Protein gm
🕒 TOTAL							
Daily Total							
Daily Target							

Ketone Levels (mM)
0   0.5   1.0   1.5   2.0   2.5   3.0   5.0+

Fasting Clock
Fast start _____
Fast finish _____
Hours fasted ☐

Exercise notes
What _____
Duration _____
Calories Burned _____

Vitamins / Supplements / Meds.

Description	Qty

How was today?

_____

_____

WEEKLY WINS

What went well this week? What can I take forward to next week?

Making next week even better

What have you learned this week? What could have been better?

_____

_____

_____

_____

_____

_____

What can you implement next week to ensure success?

_____

_____

_____

_____

_____

_____

Do not forget to record any measurements you wish to track weekly in the reference section.

"MOTIVATE THE MIND AND THE BODY WILL FOLLOW"

WEEK OF ____

Date: _____   Mon. Tue. Wed. Thur. Fri. Sat. Sun.

BREAKFAST	Amount	Cal.	Fat gm	Carb. gm	Fiber gm	Net Carb. gm	Protein gm
TOTAL							

SNACK	Amount	Cal.	Fat gm	Carb. gm	Fiber gm	Net Carb. gm	Protein gm
TOTAL							

LUNCH	Amount	Cal.	Fat gm	Carb. gm	Fiber gm	Net Carb. gm	Protein gm
TOTAL							

SNACK	Amount	Cal.	Fat gm	Carb. gm	Fiber gm	Net Carb. gm	Protein gm
TOTAL							

        8 oz

Step 2 – Tracking Food

DINNER	Amount	Cal.	Fat gm	Carb. gm	Fiber gm	Net Carb. gm	Protein gm
🕒 TOTAL							

SNACK	Amount	Cal.	Fat gm	Carb. gm	Fiber gm	Net Carb. gm	Protein gm
🕒 TOTAL							

| Daily Total | | | | | | | |
| Daily Target | | | | | | | |

Ketone Levels (mM)

|—+—+—+—+—+—+—|
0   0.5 1.0 1.5 2.0 2.5 3.0   5.0+

Fasting Clock

Fast start _____

Fast finish _____

Hours fasted ☐

Exercise notes

What _____

Duration _____

Calories Burned _____

Vitamins / Supplements / Meds.

Description	Qty

How was today?

_____

_____

DAILY

Date: _____ Mon. Tue. Wed. Thur. Fri. Sat. Sun.

BREAKFAST	Amount	Cal.	Fat gm	Carb. gm	Fiber gm	Net Carb. gm	Protein gm
🕐 TOTAL							

SNACK	Amount	Cal.	Fat gm	Carb. gm	Fiber gm	Net Carb. gm	Protein gm
🕐 TOTAL							

LUNCH	Amount	Cal.	Fat gm	Carb. gm	Fiber gm	Net Carb. gm	Protein gm
🕐 TOTAL							

SNACK	Amount	Cal.	Fat gm	Carb. gm	Fiber gm	Net Carb. gm	Protein gm
🕐 TOTAL							

🥛 🥛 🥛 🥛 🥛 🥛 🥛 🥛 8 oz

Step 2 – Tracking Food

DINNER	Amount	Cal.	Fat gm	Carb. gm	Fiber gm	Net Carb. gm	Protein gm
TOTAL							

SNACK	Amount	Cal.	Fat gm	Carb. gm	Fiber gm	Net Carb. gm	Protein gm
TOTAL							

| Daily Total | | | | | | | |
| Daily Target | | | | | | | |

Ketone Levels (mM)

0   0.5   1.0   1.5   2.0   2.5   3.0   5.0+

Fasting Clock

Fast start _____

Fast finish _____

Hours fasted ⬜

Exercise notes

What _____

Duration _____

Calories Burned _____

Vitamins / Supplements / Meds.

Description	Qty

How was today?

_____

_____

DAILY

Date: Mon.   Tue.   Wed.   Thur.   Fri.   Sat.   Sun.

BREAKFAST	Amount	Cal.	Fat gm	Carb. gm	Fiber gm	Net Carb. gm	Protein gm
🕐 TOTAL							

SNACK	Amount	Cal.	Fat gm	Carb. gm	Fiber gm	Net Carb. gm	Protein gm
🕐 TOTAL							

LUNCH	Amount	Cal.	Fat gm	Carb. gm	Fiber gm	Net Carb. gm	Protein gm
🕐 TOTAL							

SNACK	Amount	Cal.	Fat gm	Carb. gm	Fiber gm	Net Carb. gm	Protein gm
🕐 TOTAL							

8 oz

Step 2 – Tracking Food

DINNER	Amount	Cal.	Fat gm	Carb. gm	Fiber gm	Net Carb. gm	Protein gm
⏲ TOTAL							

SNACK	Amount	Cal.	Fat gm	Carb. gm	Fiber gm	Net Carb. gm	Protein gm
⏲ TOTAL							
Daily Total							
Daily Target							

Ketone Levels (mM)

├──┼──┼──┼──┼──┼──┤
0   0.5 1.0 1.5 2.0 2.5 3.0   5.0+

Fasting Clock

Fast start _____   Hours fasted

Fast finish _____

Exercise notes

What _____

Duration _____

Calories Burned _____

Vitamins / Supplements / Meds.

Description	Qty

How was today?

_____

_____

_____

DAILY

Date: Mon. Tue. Wed. Thur. Fri. Sat. Sun.

BREAKFAST	Amount	Cal.	Fat gm	Carb. gm	Fiber gm	Net Carb. gm	Protein gm
TOTAL							

SNACK	Amount	Cal.	Fat gm	Carb. gm	Fiber gm	Net Carb. gm	Protein gm
TOTAL							

LUNCH	Amount	Cal.	Fat gm	Carb. gm	Fiber gm	Net Carb. gm	Protein gm
TOTAL							

SNACK	Amount	Cal.	Fat gm	Carb. gm	Fiber gm	Net Carb. gm	Protein gm
TOTAL							

8 oz

Step 2 – Tracking Food

DINNER	Amount	Cal.	Fat gm	Carb. gm	Fiber gm	Net Carb. gm	Protein gm
⏲ TOTAL							

SNACK	Amount	Cal.	Fat gm	Carb. gm	Fiber gm	Net Carb. gm	Protein gm
⏲ TOTAL							

| Daily Total | | | | | | | |
| Daily Target | | | | | | | |

Ketone Levels (mM)

|—|—|—|—|—|—|—|
0   0.5   1.0   1.5   2.0   2.5   3.0   5.0+

Fasting Clock

Fast start _____   Hours fasted

Fast finish _____

Exercise notes

What _____

Duration _____

Calories Burned _____

Vitamins / Supplements / Meds.

Description	Qty

How was today?

_____

_____

_____

DAILY

Date: _____ Mon. Tue. Wed. Thur. Fri. Sat. Sun.

BREAKFAST	Amount	Cal.	Fat gm	Carb. gm	Fiber gm	Net Carb. gm	Protein gm
🕐 TOTAL							

SNACK	Amount	Cal.	Fat gm	Carb. gm	Fiber gm	Net Carb. gm	Protein gm
🕐 TOTAL							

LUNCH	Amount	Cal.	Fat gm	Carb. gm	Fiber gm	Net Carb. gm	Protein gm
🕐 TOTAL							

SNACK	Amount	Cal.	Fat gm	Carb. gm	Fiber gm	Net Carb. gm	Protein gm
🕐 TOTAL							

8 oz

Step 2 – Tracking Food

DINNER	Amount	Cal.	Fat gm	Carb. gm	Fiber gm	Net Carb. gm	Protein gm
TOTAL							

SNACK	Amount	Cal.	Fat gm	Carb. gm	Fiber gm	Net Carb. gm	Protein gm
TOTAL							

| Daily Total | | | | | | | |
| Daily Target | | | | | | | |

Ketone Levels (mM)

0   0.5   1.0   1.5   2.0   2.5   3.0   5.0+

Fasting Clock
Fast start _____
Fast finish _____

Hours fasted

Exercise notes
What _____
Duration _____
Calories Burned _____

Vitamins / Supplements / Meds.

Description	Qty

How was today?

_____

_____

_____

DAILY

Date: Mon.   Tue.   Wed.   Thur.   Fri.   Sat.   Sun.

BREAKFAST	Amount	Cal.	Fat gm	Carb. gm	Fiber gm	Net Carb. gm	Protein gm
🕐 TOTAL							

SNACK	Amount	Cal.	Fat gm	Carb. gm	Fiber gm	Net Carb. gm	Protein gm
🕐 TOTAL							

LUNCH	Amount	Cal.	Fat gm	Carb. gm	Fiber gm	Net Carb. gm	Protein gm
🕐 TOTAL							

SNACK	Amount	Cal.	Fat gm	Carb. gm	Fiber gm	Net Carb. gm	Protein gm
🕐 TOTAL							

        8 oz

Step 2 – Tracking Food

DINNER	Amount	Cal.	Fat gm	Carb. gm	Fiber gm	Net Carb. gm	Protein gm
TOTAL							

SNACK	Amount	Cal.	Fat gm	Carb. gm	Fiber gm	Net Carb. gm	Protein gm
TOTAL							

Daily Total							
Daily Target							

Ketone Levels (mM)

0   0.5   1.0   1.5   2.0   2.5   3.0   5.0+

Fasting Clock

Fast start _____   Hours fasted

Fast finish _____

Exercise notes

What _____

Duration _____

Calories Burned _____

Vitamins / Supplements / Meds.

Description	Qty

How was today?

_____

_____

_____

DAILY

Date: Mon. Tue. Wed. Thur. Fri. Sat. Sun.

BREAKFAST	Amount	Cal.	Fat gm	Carb. gm	Fiber gm	Net Carb. gm	Protein gm
⏲ TOTAL							

SNACK	Amount	Cal.	Fat gm	Carb. gm	Fiber gm	Net Carb. gm	Protein gm
⏲ TOTAL							

LUNCH	Amount	Cal.	Fat gm	Carb. gm	Fiber gm	Net Carb. gm	Protein gm
⏲ TOTAL							

SNACK	Amount	Cal.	Fat gm	Carb. gm	Fiber gm	Net Carb. gm	Protein gm
⏲ TOTAL							

        8 oz

Step 2 – Tracking Food

DINNER	Amount	Cal.	Fat gm	Carb. gm	Fiber gm	Net Carb. gm	Protein gm
TOTAL							

SNACK	Amount	Cal.	Fat gm	Carb. gm	Fiber gm	Net Carb. gm	Protein gm
TOTAL							

| Daily Total | | | | | | | |
| Daily Target | | | | | | | |

Ketone Levels (mM)

0   0.5   1.0   1.5   2.0   2.5   3.0   5.0+

Fasting Clock

Fast start _____   Hours fasted

Fast finish _____

Exercise notes

What _____

Duration _____

Calories Burned _____

Vitamins / Supplements / Meds.

Description	Qty

How was today?

_____

_____

WEEKLY WINS

What went well this week? What can I take forward to next week?

Making next week even better

What have you learned this week? What could have been better?

_____

_____

_____

_____

_____

_____

What can you implement next week to ensure success?

_____

_____

_____

_____

_____

_____

Do not forget to record any measurements you wish to track weekly in the reference section.

> **"YOU ARE WHAT YOU EAT. WHAT WOULD YOU LIKE TO BE TODAY?"**

WEEK OF ____

Date:				Mon.	Tue.	Wed.	Thur.	Fri.	Sat.	Sun.
BREAKFAST			Amount	Cal.	Fat gm	Carb. gm	Fiber gm	Net Carb. gm	Protein gm	
🕐		TOTAL								
SNACK			Amount	Cal.	Fat gm	Carb. gm	Fiber gm	Net Carb. gm	Protein gm	
🕐		TOTAL								
LUNCH			Amount	Cal.	Fat gm	Carb. gm	Fiber gm	Net Carb. gm	Protein gm	
🕐		TOTAL								
SNACK			Amount	Cal.	Fat gm	Carb. gm	Fiber gm	Net Carb. gm	Protein gm	
🕐		TOTAL								

        8 oz

Step 2 – Tracking Food

DINNER	Amount	Cal.	Fat gm	Carb. gm	Fiber gm	Net Carb. gm	Protein gm
TOTAL							

SNACK	Amount	Cal.	Fat gm	Carb. gm	Fiber gm	Net Carb. gm	Protein gm
TOTAL							
Daily Total							
Daily Target							

Ketone Levels (mM)
0   0.5   1.0   1.5   2.0   2.5   3.0   5.0+

Fasting Clock
Fast start _____   Hours fasted
Fast finish _____

Exercise notes
What _____
Duration _____
Calories Burned _____

Vitamins / Supplements / Meds.

Description	Qty

How was today?
_____
_____
_____

DAILY

Date: Mon.   Tue.   Wed.   Thur.   Fri.   Sat.   Sun.

BREAKFAST	Amount	Cal.	Fat gm	Carb. gm	Fiber gm	Net Carb. gm	Protein gm
TOTAL							

SNACK	Amount	Cal.	Fat gm	Carb. gm	Fiber gm	Net Carb. gm	Protein gm
TOTAL							

LUNCH	Amount	Cal.	Fat gm	Carb. gm	Fiber gm	Net Carb. gm	Protein gm
TOTAL							

SNACK	Amount	Cal.	Fat gm	Carb. gm	Fiber gm	Net Carb. gm	Protein gm
TOTAL							

8 oz

Step 2 – Tracking Food

DINNER	Amount	Cal.	Fat gm	Carb. gm	Fiber gm	Net Carb. gm	Protein gm
TOTAL							

SNACK	Amount	Cal.	Fat gm	Carb. gm	Fiber gm	Net Carb. gm	Protein gm
TOTAL							

Daily Total						
Daily Target						

Ketone Levels (mM)

0   0.5   1.0   1.5   2.0   2.5   3.0   5.0+

Fasting Clock

Fast start _____   Hours fasted

Fast finish _____

Exercise notes

What _____

Duration _____

Calories Burned _____

Vitamins / Supplements / Meds.

Description	Qty

How was today?

_____

_____

DAILY

Date: _____   Mon. Tue. Wed. Thur. Fri. Sat. Sun.

BREAKFAST	Amount	Cal.	Fat gm	Carb. gm	Fiber gm	Net Carb. gm	Protein gm
🕐 TOTAL							

SNACK	Amount	Cal.	Fat gm	Carb. gm	Fiber gm	Net Carb. gm	Protein gm
🕐 TOTAL							

LUNCH	Amount	Cal.	Fat gm	Carb. gm	Fiber gm	Net Carb. gm	Protein gm
🕐 TOTAL							

SNACK	Amount	Cal.	Fat gm	Carb. gm	Fiber gm	Net Carb. gm	Protein gm
🕐 TOTAL							

 8 oz

Step 2 – Tracking Food

DINNER	Amount	Cal.	Fat gm	Carb. gm	Fiber gm	Net Carb. gm	Protein gm
TOTAL							

SNACK	Amount	Cal.	Fat gm	Carb. gm	Fiber gm	Net Carb. gm	Protein gm
TOTAL							

| Daily Total |
| Daily Target |

Ketone Levels (mM)
0   0.5   1.0   1.5   2.0   2.5   3.0   5.0+

Fasting Clock
Fast start _____
Fast finish _____
Hours fasted

Exercise notes
What _____
Duration _____
Calories Burned _____

Vitamins / Supplements / Meds.

Description	Qty

How was today?
_____
_____

DAILY

Date: Mon.   Tue.   Wed.   Thur.   Fri.   Sat.   Sun.

BREAKFAST	Amount	Cal.	Fat gm	Carb. gm	Fiber gm	Net Carb. gm	Protein gm
TOTAL							

SNACK	Amount	Cal.	Fat gm	Carb. gm	Fiber gm	Net Carb. gm	Protein gm
TOTAL							

LUNCH	Amount	Cal.	Fat gm	Carb. gm	Fiber gm	Net Carb. gm	Protein gm
TOTAL							

SNACK	Amount	Cal.	Fat gm	Carb. gm	Fiber gm	Net Carb. gm	Protein gm
TOTAL							

8 oz

Step 2 – Tracking Food

DINNER	Amount	Cal.	Fat gm	Carb. gm	Fiber gm	Net Carb. gm	Protein gm
🕐 TOTAL							

SNACK	Amount	Cal.	Fat gm	Carb. gm	Fiber gm	Net Carb. gm	Protein gm
🕐 TOTAL							

| Daily Total | | | | | | | |
| Daily Target | | | | | | | |

Ketone Levels (mM)

├──┼──┼──┼──┼──┼──┤
0   0.5 1.0 1.5 2.0 2.5 3.0   5.0+

Fasting Clock

Fast start _____   Hours fasted

Fast finish _____   [   ]

Exercise notes

What _____

Duration _____

Calories Burned _____

Vitamins / Supplements / Meds.

Description	Qty

How was today?

_____

_____

DAILY

Date: Mon. Tue. Wed. Thur. Fri. Sat. Sun.

BREAKFAST	Amount	Cal.	Fat gm	Carb. gm	Fiber gm	Net Carb. gm	Protein gm
⊙ TOTAL							

SNACK	Amount	Cal.	Fat gm	Carb. gm	Fiber gm	Net Carb. gm	Protein gm
⊙ TOTAL							

LUNCH	Amount	Cal.	Fat gm	Carb. gm	Fiber gm	Net Carb. gm	Protein gm
⊙ TOTAL							

SNACK	Amount	Cal.	Fat gm	Carb. gm	Fiber gm	Net Carb. gm	Protein gm
⊙ TOTAL							

8 oz

Step 2 – Tracking Food

DINNER	Amount	Cal.	Fat gm	Carb. gm	Fiber gm	Net Carb. gm	Protein gm
TOTAL							

SNACK	Amount	Cal.	Fat gm	Carb. gm	Fiber gm	Net Carb. gm	Protein gm
TOTAL							

| Daily Total | | | | | | | |
| Daily Target | | | | | | | |

Ketone Levels (mM)

0   0.5   1.0   1.5   2.0   2.5   3.0   5.0+

Fasting Clock

Fast start _____

Fast finish _____

Hours fasted

Exercise notes

What _____

Duration _____

Calories Burned _____

Vitamins / Supplements / Meds.

Description	Qty

How was today?

_____

_____

DAILY

Date: _____ Mon. Tue. Wed. Thur. Fri. Sat. Sun.

BREAKFAST	Amount	Cal.	Fat gm	Carb. gm	Fiber gm	Net Carb. gm	Protein gm
🕐 TOTAL							

SNACK	Amount	Cal.	Fat gm	Carb. gm	Fiber gm	Net Carb. gm	Protein gm
🕐 TOTAL							

LUNCH	Amount	Cal.	Fat gm	Carb. gm	Fiber gm	Net Carb. gm	Protein gm
🕐 TOTAL							

SNACK	Amount	Cal.	Fat gm	Carb. gm	Fiber gm	Net Carb. gm	Protein gm
🕐 TOTAL							

8 oz

Step 2 – Tracking Food

DINNER	Amount	Cal.	Fat gm	Carb. gm	Fiber gm	Net Carb. gm	Protein gm
TOTAL							

SNACK	Amount	Cal.	Fat gm	Carb. gm	Fiber gm	Net Carb. gm	Protein gm
TOTAL							

| Daily Total | | | | | | | |
| Daily Target | | | | | | | |

Ketone Levels (mM)

0 0.5 1.0 1.5 2.0 2.5 3.0 5.0+

Fasting Clock
Fast start _____
Fast finish _____
Hours fasted _____

Exercise notes
What _____
Duration _____
Calories Burned _____

Vitamins / Supplements / Meds.

Description	Qty

How was today?
_____
_____

DAILY

Date: _____ Mon. Tue. Wed. Thur. Fri. Sat. Sun.

BREAKFAST	Amount	Cal.	Fat gm	Carb. gm	Fiber gm	Net Carb. gm	Protein gm
🕐 TOTAL							

SNACK	Amount	Cal.	Fat gm	Carb. gm	Fiber gm	Net Carb. gm	Protein gm
🕐 TOTAL							

LUNCH	Amount	Cal.	Fat gm	Carb. gm	Fiber gm	Net Carb. gm	Protein gm
🕐 TOTAL							

SNACK	Amount	Cal.	Fat gm	Carb. gm	Fiber gm	Net Carb. gm	Protein gm
🕐 TOTAL							

🥛 🥛 🥛 🥛 🥛 🥛 🥛 🥛 8 oz

Step 2 – Tracking Food

DINNER	Amount	Cal.	Fat gm	Carb. gm	Fiber gm	Net Carb. gm	Protein gm
TOTAL							

SNACK	Amount	Cal.	Fat gm	Carb. gm	Fiber gm	Net Carb. gm	Protein gm
TOTAL							

| Daily Total | | | | | | | |
| Daily Target | | | | | | | |

Ketone Levels (mM)

|—|—|—|—|—|—|—|
0   0.5   1.0   1.5   2.0   2.5   3.0   5.0+

Fasting Clock

Fast start _____   Hours fasted

Fast finish _____

Exercise notes

What _____

Duration _____

Calories Burned _____

Vitamins / Supplements / Meds.

Description	Qty

How was today?

_____

_____

WEEKLY WINS

What went well this week? What can I take forward to next week?

Making next week even better

What have you learned this week? What could have been better?

_____

_____

_____

_____

_____

What can you implement next week to ensure success?

_____

_____

_____

_____

_____

Do not forget to record any measurements you wish to track weekly in the reference section.

> **"YOUR LIFE DOES NOT GET BETTER BY CHANCE, IT GETS BETTER BY CHANGE"**

WEEK OF ___

Date: _____   Mon. Tue. Wed. Thur. Fri. Sat. Sun.

BREAKFAST	Amount	Cal.	Fat gm	Carb. gm	Fiber gm	Net Carb. gm	Protein gm
🕐 TOTAL							

SNACK	Amount	Cal.	Fat gm	Carb. gm	Fiber gm	Net Carb. gm	Protein gm
🕐 TOTAL							

LUNCH	Amount	Cal.	Fat gm	Carb. gm	Fiber gm	Net Carb. gm	Protein gm
🕐 TOTAL							

SNACK	Amount	Cal.	Fat gm	Carb. gm	Fiber gm	Net Carb. gm	Protein gm
🕐 TOTAL							

🥛 🥛 🥛 🥛 🥛 🥛 🥛 🥛   8 oz

Step 2 – Tracking Food

DINNER	Amount	Cal.	Fat gm	Carb. gm	Fiber gm	Net Carb. gm	Protein gm
TOTAL							

SNACK	Amount	Cal.	Fat gm	Carb. gm	Fiber gm	Net Carb. gm	Protein gm
TOTAL							

| Daily Total | | | | | | | |
| Daily Target | | | | | | | |

Ketone Levels (mM)

|—|—|—|—|—|—|—|
0   0.5 1.0 1.5 2.0 2.5 3.0   5.0+

Fasting Clock

Fast start _____ Hours fasted ☐

Fast finish _____

Exercise notes

What _____

Duration _____

Calories Burned _____

Vitamins / Supplements / Meds.

Description	Qty

How was today?

_____

_____

DAILY

Date: _____   Mon. Tue. Wed. Thur. Fri. Sat. Sun.

BREAKFAST	Amount	Cal.	Fat gm	Carb. gm	Fiber gm	Net Carb. gm	Protein gm
🕐 TOTAL							

SNACK	Amount	Cal.	Fat gm	Carb. gm	Fiber gm	Net Carb. gm	Protein gm
🕐 TOTAL							

LUNCH	Amount	Cal.	Fat gm	Carb. gm	Fiber gm	Net Carb. gm	Protein gm
🕐 TOTAL							

SNACK	Amount	Cal.	Fat gm	Carb. gm	Fiber gm	Net Carb. gm	Protein gm
🕐 TOTAL							

🥛 🥛 🥛 🥛 🥛 🥛 🥛 🥛 8 oz

Step 2 – Tracking Food

DINNER	Amount	Cal.	Fat gm	Carb. gm	Fiber gm	Net Carb. gm	Protein gm
🕐 TOTAL							

SNACK	Amount	Cal.	Fat gm	Carb. gm	Fiber gm	Net Carb. gm	Protein gm
🕐 TOTAL							

| Daily Total | | | | | | | |
| Daily Target | | | | | | | |

Ketone Levels (mM)

├─┼─┼─┼─┼─┼─┼─┤
0   0.5 1.0 1.5 2.0 2.5 3.0   5.0+

Fasting Clock

Fast start _____   Hours fasted [   ]

Fast finish _____

Exercise notes

What _____

Duration _____

Calories Burned _____

Vitamins / Supplements / Meds.

Description	Qty

How was today?

_____

_____

DAILY

Date: _____   Mon. Tue. Wed. Thur. Fri. Sat. Sun.

BREAKFAST	Amount	Cal.	Fat gm	Carb. gm	Fiber gm	Net Carb. gm	Protein gm
🕐 TOTAL							

SNACK	Amount	Cal.	Fat gm	Carb. gm	Fiber gm	Net Carb. gm	Protein gm
🕐 TOTAL							

LUNCH	Amount	Cal.	Fat gm	Carb. gm	Fiber gm	Net Carb. gm	Protein gm
🕐 TOTAL							

SNACK	Amount	Cal.	Fat gm	Carb. gm	Fiber gm	Net Carb. gm	Protein gm
🕐 TOTAL							

8 oz

Step 2 – Tracking Food

DINNER	Amount	Cal.	Fat gm	Carb. gm	Fiber gm	Net Carb. gm	Protein gm
🕒 TOTAL							

SNACK	Amount	Cal.	Fat gm	Carb. gm	Fiber gm	Net Carb. gm	Protein gm
🕒 TOTAL							

| Daily Total | | | | | | | |
| Daily Target | | | | | | | |

Ketone Levels (mM)

|—+—+—+—+—+—+—|
0   0.5   1.0   1.5   2.0   2.5   3.0   5.0+

Fasting Clock

Fast start _____   Hours fasted ____

Fast finish _____

Exercise notes

What _____

Duration _____

Calories Burned _____

Vitamins / Supplements / Meds.

Description	Qty

How was today?

_____

_____

DAILY

Date: _____   Mon. Tue. Wed. Thur. Fri. Sat. Sun.

BREAKFAST	Amount	Cal.	Fat gm	Carb. gm	Fiber gm	Net Carb. gm	Protein gm
🕒 TOTAL							

SNACK	Amount	Cal.	Fat gm	Carb. gm	Fiber gm	Net Carb. gm	Protein gm
🕒 TOTAL							

LUNCH	Amount	Cal.	Fat gm	Carb. gm	Fiber gm	Net Carb. gm	Protein gm
🕒 TOTAL							

SNACK	Amount	Cal.	Fat gm	Carb. gm	Fiber gm	Net Carb. gm	Protein gm
🕒 TOTAL							

        8 oz

Step 2 – Tracking Food

DINNER	Amount	Cal.	Fat gm	Carb. gm	Fiber gm	Net Carb. gm	Protein gm
⏱ TOTAL							

SNACK	Amount	Cal.	Fat gm	Carb. gm	Fiber gm	Net Carb. gm	Protein gm
⏱ TOTAL							

| Daily Total | | | | | | | |
| Daily Target | | | | | | | |

Ketone Levels (mM)

|—+—+—+—+—+—+—|
0   0.5 1.0 1.5 2.0 2.5 3.0   5.0+

Fasting Clock

Fast start _____   Hours fasted ☐

Fast finish _____

Exercise notes

What _____

Duration _____

Calories Burned _____

Vitamins / Supplements / Meds.

Description	Qty

How was today?

_____

_____

DAILY

Date: _____   Mon. Tue. Wed. Thur. Fri. Sat. Sun.

BREAKFAST	Amount	Cal.	Fat gm	Carb. gm	Fiber gm	Net Carb. gm	Protein gm
🕒 TOTAL							

SNACK	Amount	Cal.	Fat gm	Carb. gm	Fiber gm	Net Carb. gm	Protein gm
🕒 TOTAL							

LUNCH	Amount	Cal.	Fat gm	Carb. gm	Fiber gm	Net Carb. gm	Protein gm
🕒 TOTAL							

SNACK	Amount	Cal.	Fat gm	Carb. gm	Fiber gm	Net Carb. gm	Protein gm
🕒 TOTAL							

8 oz

Step 2 – Tracking Food

DINNER	Amount	Cal.	Fat gm	Carb. gm	Fiber gm	Net Carb. gm	Protein gm
TOTAL							

SNACK	Amount	Cal.	Fat gm	Carb. gm	Fiber gm	Net Carb. gm	Protein gm
TOTAL							
Daily Total							
Daily Target							

Ketone Levels (mM)

0   0.5   1.0   1.5   2.0   2.5   3.0   5.0+

Fasting Clock

Fast start _____

Fast finish _____

Hours fasted

Exercise notes

What _____

Duration _____

Calories Burned _____

Vitamins / Supplements / Meds.

Description	Qty

How was today?

_____

_____

_____

DAILY

Date: _____ Mon. Tue. Wed. Thur. Fri. Sat. Sun.

BREAKFAST	Amount	Cal.	Fat gm	Carb. gm	Fiber gm	Net Carb. gm	Protein gm
⊘ TOTAL							

SNACK	Amount	Cal.	Fat gm	Carb. gm	Fiber gm	Net Carb. gm	Protein gm
⊘ TOTAL							

LUNCH	Amount	Cal.	Fat gm	Carb. gm	Fiber gm	Net Carb. gm	Protein gm
⊘ TOTAL							

SNACK	Amount	Cal.	Fat gm	Carb. gm	Fiber gm	Net Carb. gm	Protein gm
⊘ TOTAL							

🥛 🥛 🥛 🥛 🥛 🥛 🥛 🥛 8 oz

Step 2 – Tracking Food

DINNER	Amount	Cal.	Fat gm	Carb. gm	Fiber gm	Net Carb. gm	Protein gm
TOTAL							

SNACK	Amount	Cal.	Fat gm	Carb. gm	Fiber gm	Net Carb. gm	Protein gm
TOTAL							

| Daily Total | | | | | | | |
| Daily Target | | | | | | | |

Ketone Levels (mM)
0   0.5   1.0   1.5   2.0   2.5   3.0   5.0+

Fasting Clock
Fast start _____
Fast finish _____

Hours fasted

Exercise notes
What _____
Duration _____
Calories Burned _____

Vitamins / Supplements / Meds.

Description	Qty

How was today?

_____
_____

DAILY

Date: _____ Mon. Tue. Wed. Thur. Fri. Sat. Sun.

BREAKFAST	Amount	Cal.	Fat gm	Carb. gm	Fiber gm	Net Carb. gm	Protein gm
⊘ TOTAL							

SNACK	Amount	Cal.	Fat gm	Carb. gm	Fiber gm	Net Carb. gm	Protein gm
⊘ TOTAL							

LUNCH	Amount	Cal.	Fat gm	Carb. gm	Fiber gm	Net Carb. gm	Protein gm
⊘ TOTAL							

SNACK	Amount	Cal.	Fat gm	Carb. gm	Fiber gm	Net Carb. gm	Protein gm
⊘ TOTAL							

8 oz

Step 2 – Tracking Food

DINNER	Amount	Cal.	Fat gm	Carb. gm	Fiber gm	Net Carb. gm	Protein gm
🕐 TOTAL							

SNACK	Amount	Cal.	Fat gm	Carb. gm	Fiber gm	Net Carb. gm	Protein gm
🕐 TOTAL							
Daily Total							
Daily Target							

Ketone Levels (mM)

| 0 | 0.5 | 1.0 | 1.5 | 2.0 | 2.5 | 3.0 | 5.0+ |

Fasting Clock

Fast start _____   Hours fasted _____

Fast finish _____

Exercise notes

What _____

Duration _____

Calories Burned _____

Vitamins / Supplements / Meds.

Description	Qty

How was today?

_____

_____

WEEKLY WINS

What went well this week? What can I take forward to next week?

Making next week even better

What have you learned this week? What could have been better?

_____
_____
_____
_____
_____
_____
_____

What can you implement next week to ensure success?

_____
_____
_____
_____
_____
_____
_____

Do not forget to record any measurements you wish to track weekly in the reference section.

"THE GREATEST WEALTH IS YOUR HEALTH"

WEEK OF ____

Date: Mon.   Tue.   Wed.   Thur.   Fri.   Sat.   Sun.

BREAKFAST	Amount	Cal.	Fat gm	Carb. gm	Fiber gm	Net Carb. gm	Protein gm
TOTAL							

SNACK	Amount	Cal.	Fat gm	Carb. gm	Fiber gm	Net Carb. gm	Protein gm
TOTAL							

LUNCH	Amount	Cal.	Fat gm	Carb. gm	Fiber gm	Net Carb. gm	Protein gm
TOTAL							

SNACK	Amount	Cal.	Fat gm	Carb. gm	Fiber gm	Net Carb. gm	Protein gm
TOTAL							

      8 oz

Step 2 – Tracking Food

DINNER	Amount	Cal.	Fat gm	Carb. gm	Fiber gm	Net Carb. gm	Protein gm
TOTAL							

SNACK	Amount	Cal.	Fat gm	Carb. gm	Fiber gm	Net Carb. gm	Protein gm
TOTAL							

| Daily Total | | | | | | | |
| Daily Target | | | | | | | |

Ketone Levels (mM)

0   0.5   1.0   1.5   2.0   2.5   3.0   5.0+

Fasting Clock

Fast start _____   Hours fasted ⬚

Fast finish _____

Exercise notes

What _____

Duration _____

Calories Burned _____

Vitamins / Supplements / Meds.

Description	Qty

How was today?

_____

_____

DAILY

Date: _____   Mon. Tue. Wed. Thur. Fri. Sat. Sun.

BREAKFAST	Amount	Cal.	Fat gm	Carb. gm	Fiber gm	Net Carb. gm	Protein gm
🕐 TOTAL							

SNACK	Amount	Cal.	Fat gm	Carb. gm	Fiber gm	Net Carb. gm	Protein gm
🕐 TOTAL							

LUNCH	Amount	Cal.	Fat gm	Carb. gm	Fiber gm	Net Carb. gm	Protein gm
🕐 TOTAL							

SNACK	Amount	Cal.	Fat gm	Carb. gm	Fiber gm	Net Carb. gm	Protein gm
🕐 TOTAL							

8 oz

Step 2 – Tracking Food

DINNER	Amount	Cal.	Fat gm	Carb. gm	Fiber gm	Net Carb. gm	Protein gm
TOTAL							

SNACK	Amount	Cal.	Fat gm	Carb. gm	Fiber gm	Net Carb. gm	Protein gm
TOTAL							

| Daily Total | | | | | | | |
| Daily Target | | | | | | | |

Ketone Levels (mM)

0   0.5   1.0   1.5   2.0   2.5   3.0   5.0+

Fasting Clock

Fast start _____   Hours fasted

Fast finish _____

Exercise notes

What _____

Duration _____

Calories Burned _____

Vitamins / Supplements / Meds.

Description	Qty

How was today?

_____

_____

DAILY

Date: _____   Mon. Tue. Wed. Thur. Fri. Sat. Sun.

BREAKFAST	Amount	Cal.	Fat gm	Carb. gm	Fiber gm	Net Carb. gm	Protein gm
🕐 TOTAL							

SNACK	Amount	Cal.	Fat gm	Carb. gm	Fiber gm	Net Carb. gm	Protein gm
🕐 TOTAL							

LUNCH	Amount	Cal.	Fat gm	Carb. gm	Fiber gm	Net Carb. gm	Protein gm
🕐 TOTAL							

SNACK	Amount	Cal.	Fat gm	Carb. gm	Fiber gm	Net Carb. gm	Protein gm
🕐 TOTAL							

8 oz

Step 2 – Tracking Food

DINNER	Amount	Cal.	Fat gm	Carb. gm	Fiber gm	Net Carb. gm	Protein gm
TOTAL							

SNACK	Amount	Cal.	Fat gm	Carb. gm	Fiber gm	Net Carb. gm	Protein gm
TOTAL							

| Daily Total | | | | | | | |
| Daily Target | | | | | | | |

Ketone Levels (mM)
0   0.5   1.0   1.5   2.0   2.5   3.0   5.0+

Fasting Clock
Fast start _____   Hours fasted
Fast finish _____

Exercise notes
What _____
Duration _____
Calories Burned _____

Vitamins / Supplements / Meds.

Description	Qty

How was today?

_____
_____
_____

DAILY

Date: _____   Mon. Tue. Wed. Thur. Fri. Sat. Sun.

BREAKFAST	Amount	Cal.	Fat gm	Carb. gm	Fiber gm	Net Carb. gm	Protein gm
🕐 TOTAL							

SNACK	Amount	Cal.	Fat gm	Carb. gm	Fiber gm	Net Carb. gm	Protein gm
🕐 TOTAL							

LUNCH	Amount	Cal.	Fat gm	Carb. gm	Fiber gm	Net Carb. gm	Protein gm
🕐 TOTAL							

SNACK	Amount	Cal.	Fat gm	Carb. gm	Fiber gm	Net Carb. gm	Protein gm
🕐 TOTAL							

        8 oz

Step 2 – Tracking Food

DINNER	Amount	Cal.	Fat gm	Carb. gm	Fiber gm	Net Carb. gm	Protein gm
⏲ TOTAL							

SNACK	Amount	Cal.	Fat gm	Carb. gm	Fiber gm	Net Carb. gm	Protein gm
⏲ TOTAL							

| Daily Total | | | | | | | |
| Daily Target | | | | | | | |

Ketone Levels (mM)

├──┼──┼──┼──┼──┤
0   0.5   1.0   1.5   2.0   2.5   3.0   5.0+

Fasting Clock
Fast start _____   Hours fasted
Fast finish _____

Exercise notes
What _____
Duration _____
Calories Burned _____

Vitamins / Supplements / Meds.

Description	Qty

How was today?
_____
_____

DAILY

Date: _____   Mon. Tue. Wed. Thur. Fri. Sat. Sun.

BREAKFAST	Amount	Cal.	Fat gm	Carb. gm	Fiber gm	Net Carb. gm	Protein gm
⊙ TOTAL							

SNACK	Amount	Cal.	Fat gm	Carb. gm	Fiber gm	Net Carb. gm	Protein gm
⊙ TOTAL							

LUNCH	Amount	Cal.	Fat gm	Carb. gm	Fiber gm	Net Carb. gm	Protein gm
⊙ TOTAL							

SNACK	Amount	Cal.	Fat gm	Carb. gm	Fiber gm	Net Carb. gm	Protein gm
⊙ TOTAL							

        8 oz

Step 2 – Tracking Food

DINNER	Amount	Cal.	Fat gm	Carb. gm	Fiber gm	Net Carb. gm	Protein gm
TOTAL							

SNACK	Amount	Cal.	Fat gm	Carb. gm	Fiber gm	Net Carb. gm	Protein gm
TOTAL							

| Daily Total | | | | | | | |
| Daily Target | | | | | | | |

Ketone Levels (mM)

0   0.5   1.0   1.5   2.0   2.5   3.0   5.0+

Fasting Clock
Fast start _____
Fast finish _____
Hours fasted _____

Exercise notes
What _____
Duration _____
Calories Burned _____

Vitamins / Supplements / Meds.

Description	Qty

How was today?

_____
_____

DAILY

Date: _____ Mon. Tue. Wed. Thur. Fri. Sat. Sun.

BREAKFAST	Amount	Cal.	Fat gm	Carb. gm	Fiber gm	Net Carb. gm	Protein gm
🕐 TOTAL							

SNACK	Amount	Cal.	Fat gm	Carb. gm	Fiber gm	Net Carb. gm	Protein gm
🕐 TOTAL							

LUNCH	Amount	Cal.	Fat gm	Carb. gm	Fiber gm	Net Carb. gm	Protein gm
🕐 TOTAL							

SNACK	Amount	Cal.	Fat gm	Carb. gm	Fiber gm	Net Carb. gm	Protein gm
🕐 TOTAL							

8 oz

Step 2 – Tracking Food

DINNER	Amount	Cal.	Fat gm	Carb. gm	Fiber gm	Net Carb. gm	Protein gm
TOTAL							

SNACK	Amount	Cal.	Fat gm	Carb. gm	Fiber gm	Net Carb. gm	Protein gm
TOTAL							
Daily Total							
Daily Target							

Ketone Levels (mM)

0   0.5   1.0   1.5   2.0   2.5   3.0   5.0+

Fasting Clock
Fast start _____
Fast finish _____
Hours fasted ☐

Exercise notes
What _____
Duration _____
Calories Burned _____

Vitamins / Supplements / Meds.

Description	Qty

How was today?

_____
_____

DAILY

Date: _____ Mon. Tue. Wed. Thur. Fri. Sat. Sun.

BREAKFAST	Amount	Cal.	Fat gm	Carb. gm	Fiber gm	Net Carb. gm	Protein gm
🕐 TOTAL							

SNACK	Amount	Cal.	Fat gm	Carb. gm	Fiber gm	Net Carb. gm	Protein gm
🕐 TOTAL							

LUNCH	Amount	Cal.	Fat gm	Carb. gm	Fiber gm	Net Carb. gm	Protein gm
🕐 TOTAL							

SNACK	Amount	Cal.	Fat gm	Carb. gm	Fiber gm	Net Carb. gm	Protein gm
🕐 TOTAL							

8 oz

Step 2 – Tracking Food

DINNER	Amount	Cal.	Fat gm	Carb. gm	Fiber gm	Net Carb. gm	Protein gm
TOTAL							

SNACK	Amount	Cal.	Fat gm	Carb. gm	Fiber gm	Net Carb. gm	Protein gm
TOTAL							
Daily Total							
Daily Target							

Ketone Levels (mM)
0   0.5   1.0   1.5   2.0   2.5   3.0   5.0+

Fasting Clock
Fast start _____
Fast finish _____
Hours fasted

Exercise notes
What _____
Duration _____
Calories Burned _____

Vitamins / Supplements / Meds.

Description	Qty

How was today?
_____
_____

WEEKLY WINS

What went well this week? What can I take forward to next week?

Making next week even better

What have you learned this week? What could have been better?

_____

_____

_____

_____

_____

_____

What can you implement next week to ensure success?

_____

_____

_____

_____

_____

_____

Do not forget to record any measurements you wish to track weekly in the reference section.

"TODAY, I AM GOING TO TREAT YOU WELL. (NOTE TO SELF)"

WEEK OF ____

Date: Mon.   Tue.   Wed.   Thur.   Fri.   Sat.   Sun.

BREAKFAST	Amount	Cal.	Fat gm	Carb. gm	Fiber gm	Net Carb. gm	Protein gm
TOTAL							

SNACK	Amount	Cal.	Fat gm	Carb. gm	Fiber gm	Net Carb. gm	Protein gm
TOTAL							

LUNCH	Amount	Cal.	Fat gm	Carb. gm	Fiber gm	Net Carb. gm	Protein gm
TOTAL							

SNACK	Amount	Cal.	Fat gm	Carb. gm	Fiber gm	Net Carb. gm	Protein gm
TOTAL							

        8 oz

Step 2 – Tracking Food

DINNER	Amount	Cal.	Fat gm	Carb. gm	Fiber gm	Net Carb. gm	Protein gm
TOTAL							

SNACK	Amount	Cal.	Fat gm	Carb. gm	Fiber gm	Net Carb. gm	Protein gm
TOTAL							

| Daily Total | | | | | | | |
| Daily Target | | | | | | | |

Ketone Levels (mM)

0   0.5   1.0   1.5   2.0   2.5   3.0   5.0+

Fasting Clock
Fast start _____
Fast finish _____

Hours fasted ☐

Exercise notes
What _____
Duration _____
Calories Burned _____

Vitamins / Supplements / Meds.

Description	Qty

How was today?
_____
_____

DAILY

Date: _____ Mon. Tue. Wed. Thur. Fri. Sat. Sun.

BREAKFAST	Amount	Cal.	Fat gm	Carb. gm	Fiber gm	Net Carb. gm	Protein gm
🕐 TOTAL							

SNACK	Amount	Cal.	Fat gm	Carb. gm	Fiber gm	Net Carb. gm	Protein gm
🕐 TOTAL							

LUNCH	Amount	Cal.	Fat gm	Carb. gm	Fiber gm	Net Carb. gm	Protein gm
🕐 TOTAL							

SNACK	Amount	Cal.	Fat gm	Carb. gm	Fiber gm	Net Carb. gm	Protein gm
🕐 TOTAL							

        8 oz

Step 2 – Tracking Food

DINNER	Amount	Cal.	Fat gm	Carb. gm	Fiber gm	Net Carb. gm	Protein gm
⏱ TOTAL							

SNACK	Amount	Cal.	Fat gm	Carb. gm	Fiber gm	Net Carb. gm	Protein gm
⏱ TOTAL							

| Daily Total | | | | | | | |
| Daily Target | | | | | | | |

Ketone Levels (mM)

|—+—+—+—+—+—|
0   0.5 1.0 1.5 2.0 2.5 3.0   5.0+

Fasting Clock

Fast start _____   Hours fasted

Fast finish _____

Exercise notes

What _____

Duration _____

Calories Burned _____

Vitamins / Supplements / Meds.

Description	Qty

How was today?

_____

_____

DAILY

Date: _____ Mon. Tue. Wed. Thur. Fri. Sat. Sun.

BREAKFAST	Amount	Cal.	Fat gm	Carb. gm	Fiber gm	Net Carb. gm	Protein gm
⏲ TOTAL							

SNACK	Amount	Cal.	Fat gm	Carb. gm	Fiber gm	Net Carb. gm	Protein gm
⏲ TOTAL							

LUNCH	Amount	Cal.	Fat gm	Carb. gm	Fiber gm	Net Carb. gm	Protein gm
⏲ TOTAL							

SNACK	Amount	Cal.	Fat gm	Carb. gm	Fiber gm	Net Carb. gm	Protein gm
⏲ TOTAL							

        8 oz

Step 2 – Tracking Food

DINNER	Amount	Cal.	Fat gm	Carb. gm	Fiber gm	Net Carb. gm	Protein gm
🕐 TOTAL							

SNACK	Amount	Cal.	Fat gm	Carb. gm	Fiber gm	Net Carb. gm	Protein gm
🕐 TOTAL							
Daily Total							
Daily Target							

Ketone Levels (mM)

|—|—|—|—|—|—|—|
0   0.5   1.0   1.5   2.0   2.5   3.0   5.0+

Fasting Clock

Fast start _____   Hours fasted _____

Fast finish _____

Exercise notes

What _____

Duration _____

Calories Burned _____

Vitamins / Supplements / Meds.

Description	Qty

How was today?

_____

_____

DAILY

Date: _____   Mon. Tue. Wed. Thur. Fri. Sat. Sun.

BREAKFAST	Amount	Cal.	Fat gm	Carb. gm	Fiber gm	Net Carb. gm	Protein gm
🕒 TOTAL							

SNACK	Amount	Cal.	Fat gm	Carb. gm	Fiber gm	Net Carb. gm	Protein gm
🕒 TOTAL							

LUNCH	Amount	Cal.	Fat gm	Carb. gm	Fiber gm	Net Carb. gm	Protein gm
🕒 TOTAL							

SNACK	Amount	Cal.	Fat gm	Carb. gm	Fiber gm	Net Carb. gm	Protein gm
🕒 TOTAL							

▽ ▽ ▽ ▽ ▽ ▽ ▽ ▽ 8 oz

Step 2 – Tracking Food

DINNER	Amount	Cal.	Fat gm	Carb. gm	Fiber gm	Net Carb. gm	Protein gm
🕒 TOTAL							

SNACK	Amount	Cal.	Fat gm	Carb. gm	Fiber gm	Net Carb. gm	Protein gm
🕒 TOTAL							

| Daily Total | | | | | | | |
| Daily Target | | | | | | | |

Ketone Levels (mM)

0   0.5   1.0   1.5   2.0   2.5   3.0   5.0+

Fasting Clock

Fast start _____

Fast finish _____

Hours fasted ▢

Exercise notes

What _____

Duration _____

Calories Burned _____

Vitamins / Supplements / Meds.

Description	Qty

How was today?

_____

_____

DAILY

Date: _____ Mon. Tue. Wed. Thur. Fri. Sat. Sun.

BREAKFAST	Amount	Cal.	Fat gm	Carb. gm	Fiber gm	Net Carb. gm	Protein gm
🕒 TOTAL							

SNACK	Amount	Cal.	Fat gm	Carb. gm	Fiber gm	Net Carb. gm	Protein gm
🕒 TOTAL							

LUNCH	Amount	Cal.	Fat gm	Carb. gm	Fiber gm	Net Carb. gm	Protein gm
🕒 TOTAL							

SNACK	Amount	Cal.	Fat gm	Carb. gm	Fiber gm	Net Carb. gm	Protein gm
🕒 TOTAL							

◻ ◻ ◻ ◻ ◻ ◻ ◻ ◻ 8 oz

Step 2 – Tracking Food

DINNER	Amount	Cal.	Fat gm	Carb. gm	Fiber gm	Net Carb. gm	Protein gm
TOTAL							

SNACK	Amount	Cal.	Fat gm	Carb. gm	Fiber gm	Net Carb. gm	Protein gm
TOTAL							

Daily Total						
Daily Target						

Ketone Levels (mM)
0   0.5   1.0   1.5   2.0   2.5   3.0   5.0+

Fasting Clock
Fast start _____   Hours fasted
Fast finish _____

Exercise notes
What _____
Duration _____
Calories Burned _____

Vitamins / Supplements / Meds.

Description	Qty

How was today?
_____
_____

DAILY

Date: _____ Mon. Tue. Wed. Thur. Fri. Sat. Sun.

BREAKFAST	Amount	Cal.	Fat gm	Carb. gm	Fiber gm	Net Carb. gm	Protein gm
⏱ TOTAL							

SNACK	Amount	Cal.	Fat gm	Carb. gm	Fiber gm	Net Carb. gm	Protein gm
⏱ TOTAL							

LUNCH	Amount	Cal.	Fat gm	Carb. gm	Fiber gm	Net Carb. gm	Protein gm
⏱ TOTAL							

SNACK	Amount	Cal.	Fat gm	Carb. gm	Fiber gm	Net Carb. gm	Protein gm
⏱ TOTAL							

        8 oz

Step 2 – Tracking Food

DINNER	Amount	Cal.	Fat gm	Carb. gm	Fiber gm	Net Carb. gm	Protein gm
TOTAL							

SNACK	Amount	Cal.	Fat gm	Carb. gm	Fiber gm	Net Carb. gm	Protein gm
TOTAL							
Daily Total							
Daily Target							

Ketone Levels (mM)

0   0.5   1.0   1.5   2.0   2.5   3.0   5.0+

Fasting Clock

Fast start _____

Fast finish _____

Hours fasted

Exercise notes

What _____

Duration _____

Calories Burned _____

Vitamins / Supplements / Meds.

Description	Qty

How was today?

_____

_____

_____

DAILY

Date: Mon.   Tue.   Wed.   Thur.   Fri.   Sat.   Sun.

BREAKFAST	Amount	Cal.	Fat gm	Carb. gm	Fiber gm	Net Carb. gm	Protein gm
⏱ TOTAL							

SNACK	Amount	Cal.	Fat gm	Carb. gm	Fiber gm	Net Carb. gm	Protein gm
⏱ TOTAL							

LUNCH	Amount	Cal.	Fat gm	Carb. gm	Fiber gm	Net Carb. gm	Protein gm
⏱ TOTAL							

SNACK	Amount	Cal.	Fat gm	Carb. gm	Fiber gm	Net Carb. gm	Protein gm
⏱ TOTAL							

8 oz

Step 2 – Tracking Food

DINNER	Amount	Cal.	Fat gm	Carb. gm	Fiber gm	Net Carb. gm	Protein gm
TOTAL							

SNACK	Amount	Cal.	Fat gm	Carb. gm	Fiber gm	Net Carb. gm	Protein gm
TOTAL							

| Daily Total | | | | | | | |
| Daily Target | | | | | | | |

Ketone Levels (mM)

0   0.5   1.0   1.5   2.0   2.5   3.0   5.0+

Fasting Clock

Fast start _____   Hours fasted

Fast finish _____

Exercise notes

What _____

Duration _____

Calories Burned _____

Vitamins / Supplements / Meds.

Description	Qty

How was today?

_____

_____

WEEKLY WINS

What went well this week? What can I take forward to next week?

Making next week even better

What have you learned this week? What could have been better?

_____

_____

_____

_____

_____

_____

What can you implement next week to ensure success?

_____

_____

_____

_____

_____

Do not forget to record any measurements you wish to track weekly in the reference section.

> **"LIVE LESS OUT OF HABIT AND MORE OUT OF INTENT"**

WEEK OF ____

Date: _____   Mon. Tue. Wed. Thur. Fri. Sat. Sun.

BREAKFAST	Amount	Cal.	Fat gm	Carb. gm	Fiber gm	Net Carb. gm	Protein gm
🕐 TOTAL							

SNACK	Amount	Cal.	Fat gm	Carb. gm	Fiber gm	Net Carb. gm	Protein gm
🕐 TOTAL							

LUNCH	Amount	Cal.	Fat gm	Carb. gm	Fiber gm	Net Carb. gm	Protein gm
🕐 TOTAL							

SNACK	Amount	Cal.	Fat gm	Carb. gm	Fiber gm	Net Carb. gm	Protein gm
🕐 TOTAL							

        8 oz

Step 2 – Tracking Food

DINNER	Amount	Cal.	Fat gm	Carb. gm	Fiber gm	Net Carb. gm	Protein gm
🕐 TOTAL							

SNACK	Amount	Cal.	Fat gm	Carb. gm	Fiber gm	Net Carb. gm	Protein gm
🕐 TOTAL							
Daily Total							
Daily Target							

Ketone Levels (mM)

| 0 | 0.5 | 1.0 | 1.5 | 2.0 | 2.5 | 3.0 | 5.0+ |

Fasting Clock

Fast start _____

Fast finish _____

Hours fasted ☐

Exercise notes

What _____

Duration _____

Calories Burned _____

Vitamins / Supplements / Meds.

Description	Qty

How was today?

_____

_____

DAILY

Date: Mon.   Tue.   Wed.   Thur.   Fri.   Sat.   Sun.

BREAKFAST	Amount	Cal.	Fat gm	Carb. gm	Fiber gm	Net Carb. gm	Protein gm
🕐 TOTAL							

SNACK	Amount	Cal.	Fat gm	Carb. gm	Fiber gm	Net Carb. gm	Protein gm
🕐 TOTAL							

LUNCH	Amount	Cal.	Fat gm	Carb. gm	Fiber gm	Net Carb. gm	Protein gm
🕐 TOTAL							

SNACK	Amount	Cal.	Fat gm	Carb. gm	Fiber gm	Net Carb. gm	Protein gm
🕐 TOTAL							

        8 oz

Step 2 – Tracking Food

DINNER	Amount	Cal.	Fat gm	Carb. gm	Fiber gm	Net Carb. gm	Protein gm
	TOTAL						

SNACK	Amount	Cal.	Fat gm	Carb. gm	Fiber gm	Net Carb. gm	Protein gm
	TOTAL						

| Daily Total | | | | | | | |
| Daily Target | | | | | | | |

Ketone Levels (mM)
0   0.5   1.0   1.5   2.0   2.5   3.0   5.0+

Fasting Clock
Fast start _____
Fast finish _____
Hours fasted [ ]

Exercise notes
What _____
Duration _____
Calories Burned _____

Vitamins / Supplements / Meds.

Description	Qty

How was today?
_____
_____
_____

DAILY

Date: _____ Mon. Tue. Wed. Thur. Fri. Sat. Sun.

BREAKFAST	Amount	Cal.	Fat gm	Carb. gm	Fiber gm	Net Carb. gm	Protein gm
🕐 TOTAL							

SNACK	Amount	Cal.	Fat gm	Carb. gm	Fiber gm	Net Carb. gm	Protein gm
🕐 TOTAL							

LUNCH	Amount	Cal.	Fat gm	Carb. gm	Fiber gm	Net Carb. gm	Protein gm
🕐 TOTAL							

SNACK	Amount	Cal.	Fat gm	Carb. gm	Fiber gm	Net Carb. gm	Protein gm
🕐 TOTAL							

8 oz

Step 2 – Tracking Food

DINNER	Amount	Cal.	Fat gm	Carb. gm	Fiber gm	Net Carb. gm	Protein gm
	TOTAL						

SNACK	Amount	Cal.	Fat gm	Carb. gm	Fiber gm	Net Carb. gm	Protein gm
	TOTAL						

Daily Total							
Daily Target							

Ketone Levels (mM)

0   0.5   1.0   1.5   2.0   2.5   3.0   5.0+

Fasting Clock
Fast start _____   Hours fasted ☐
Fast finish _____

Exercise notes
What _____
Duration _____
Calories Burned _____

Vitamins / Supplements / Meds.

Description	Qty

How was today?
_____
_____
_____

DAILY

Date: _____ Mon. Tue. Wed. Thur. Fri. Sat. Sun.

BREAKFAST	Amount	Cal.	Fat gm	Carb. gm	Fiber gm	Net Carb. gm	Protein gm
🕐 TOTAL							

SNACK	Amount	Cal.	Fat gm	Carb. gm	Fiber gm	Net Carb. gm	Protein gm
🕐 TOTAL							

LUNCH	Amount	Cal.	Fat gm	Carb. gm	Fiber gm	Net Carb. gm	Protein gm
🕐 TOTAL							

SNACK	Amount	Cal.	Fat gm	Carb. gm	Fiber gm	Net Carb. gm	Protein gm
🕐 TOTAL							

8 oz

Step 2 – Tracking Food

DINNER	Amount	Cal.	Fat gm	Carb. gm	Fiber gm	Net Carb. gm	Protein gm
TOTAL							

SNACK	Amount	Cal.	Fat gm	Carb. gm	Fiber gm	Net Carb. gm	Protein gm
TOTAL							

| Daily Total | | | | | | | |
| Daily Target | | | | | | | |

Ketone Levels (mM)

|—+—+—+—+—+—|
0 0.5 1.0 1.5 2.0 2.5 3.0 5.0+

Fasting Clock

Fast start _____   Hours fasted

Fast finish _____

Exercise notes

What _____

Duration _____

Calories Burned _____

Vitamins / Supplements / Meds.

Description	Qty

How was today?

_____

_____

DAILY

Date: _____   Mon. Tue. Wed. Thur. Fri. Sat. Sun.

BREAKFAST	Amount	Cal.	Fat gm	Carb. gm	Fiber gm	Net Carb. gm	Protein gm
⊙ TOTAL							

SNACK	Amount	Cal.	Fat gm	Carb. gm	Fiber gm	Net Carb. gm	Protein gm
⊙ TOTAL							

LUNCH	Amount	Cal.	Fat gm	Carb. gm	Fiber gm	Net Carb. gm	Protein gm
⊙ TOTAL							

SNACK	Amount	Cal.	Fat gm	Carb. gm	Fiber gm	Net Carb. gm	Protein gm
⊙ TOTAL							

▯ ▯ ▯ ▯ ▯ ▯ ▯ ▯   8 oz

Step 2 – Tracking Food

DINNER	Amount	Cal.	Fat gm	Carb. gm	Fiber gm	Net Carb. gm	Protein gm
TOTAL							

SNACK	Amount	Cal.	Fat gm	Carb. gm	Fiber gm	Net Carb. gm	Protein gm
TOTAL							

| Daily Total | | | | | | | |
| Daily Target | | | | | | | |

Ketone Levels (mM)

| 0 | 0.5 | 1.0 | 1.5 | 2.0 | 2.5 | 3.0 | 5.0+ |

Fasting Clock

Fast start _____

Fast finish _____

Hours fasted

Exercise notes

What _____

Duration _____

Calories Burned _____

Vitamins / Supplements / Meds.

Description	Qty

How was today?

_____

_____

DAILY

Date: _____   Mon. Tue. Wed. Thur. Fri. Sat. Sun.

BREAKFAST	Amount	Cal.	Fat gm	Carb. gm	Fiber gm	Net Carb. gm	Protein gm
🕐 TOTAL							

SNACK	Amount	Cal.	Fat gm	Carb. gm	Fiber gm	Net Carb. gm	Protein gm
🕐 TOTAL							

LUNCH	Amount	Cal.	Fat gm	Carb. gm	Fiber gm	Net Carb. gm	Protein gm
🕐 TOTAL							

SNACK	Amount	Cal.	Fat gm	Carb. gm	Fiber gm	Net Carb. gm	Protein gm
🕐 TOTAL							

        8 oz

Step 2 – Tracking Food

DINNER	Amount	Cal.	Fat gm	Carb. gm	Fiber gm	Net Carb. gm	Protein gm
TOTAL							

SNACK	Amount	Cal.	Fat gm	Carb. gm	Fiber gm	Net Carb. gm	Protein gm
TOTAL							

| Daily Total | | | | | | | |
| Daily Target | | | | | | | |

Ketone Levels (mM)

| 0 | 0.5 | 1.0 | 1.5 | 2.0 | 2.5 | 3.0 | 5.0+ |

Fasting Clock

Fast start _____   Hours fasted _____

Fast finish _____

Exercise notes

What _____

Duration _____

Calories Burned _____

Vitamins / Supplements / Meds.

Description	Qty

How was today?

_____

_____

DAILY

Date: _____   Mon. Tue. Wed. Thur. Fri. Sat. Sun.

BREAKFAST	Amount	Cal.	Fat gm	Carb. gm	Fiber gm	Net Carb. gm	Protein gm
🕐 TOTAL							

SNACK	Amount	Cal.	Fat gm	Carb. gm	Fiber gm	Net Carb. gm	Protein gm
🕐 TOTAL							

LUNCH	Amount	Cal.	Fat gm	Carb. gm	Fiber gm	Net Carb. gm	Protein gm
🕐 TOTAL							

SNACK	Amount	Cal.	Fat gm	Carb. gm	Fiber gm	Net Carb. gm	Protein gm
🕐 TOTAL							

8 oz

Step 2 – Tracking Food

DINNER	Amount	Cal.	Fat gm	Carb. gm	Fiber gm	Net Carb. gm	Protein gm
TOTAL							

SNACK	Amount	Cal.	Fat gm	Carb. gm	Fiber gm	Net Carb. gm	Protein gm
TOTAL							

| Daily Total | | | | | | | |
| Daily Target | | | | | | | |

Ketone Levels (mM)

0   0.5   1.0   1.5   2.0   2.5   3.0   5.0+

Fasting Clock

Fast start _____   Hours fasted ☐

Fast finish _____

Exercise notes

What _____

Duration _____

Calories Burned _____

Vitamins / Supplements / Meds.

Description	Qty

How was today?

_____

_____

WEEKLY WINS

What went well this week? What can I take forward to next week?

Making next week even better

What have you learned this week? What could have been better?

_____

_____

_____

_____

_____

_____

What can you implement next week to ensure success?

_____

_____

_____

_____

_____

_____

Do not forget to record any measurements you wish to track weekly in the reference section.

> **"IT'S NOT ABOUT BEING THE BEST, IT'S ABOUT BEING SLIGHTLY BETTER THAN YOU WERE YESTERDAY"**

WEEK OF ____

Date: Mon. Tue. Wed. Thur. Fri. Sat. Sun.

BREAKFAST	Amount	Cal.	Fat gm	Carb. gm	Fiber gm	Net Carb. gm	Protein gm
TOTAL							

SNACK	Amount	Cal.	Fat gm	Carb. gm	Fiber gm	Net Carb. gm	Protein gm
TOTAL							

LUNCH	Amount	Cal.	Fat gm	Carb. gm	Fiber gm	Net Carb. gm	Protein gm
TOTAL							

SNACK	Amount	Cal.	Fat gm	Carb. gm	Fiber gm	Net Carb. gm	Protein gm
TOTAL							

        8 oz

Step 2 – Tracking Food

DINNER	Amount	Cal.	Fat gm	Carb. gm	Fiber gm	Net Carb. gm	Protein gm
TOTAL							

SNACK	Amount	Cal.	Fat gm	Carb. gm	Fiber gm	Net Carb. gm	Protein gm
TOTAL							

| Daily Total | | | | | | | |
| Daily Target | | | | | | | |

Ketone Levels (mM)

0   0.5   1.0   1.5   2.0   2.5   3.0   5.0+

Fasting Clock

Fast start _____   Hours fasted _____

Fast finish _____

Exercise notes

What _____

Duration _____

Calories Burned _____

Vitamins / Supplements / Meds.

Description	Qty

How was today?

_____

_____

DAILY

Date: _____ Mon. Tue. Wed. Thur. Fri. Sat. Sun.

BREAKFAST	Amount	Cal.	Fat gm	Carb. gm	Fiber gm	Net Carb. gm	Protein gm
🕒 TOTAL							

SNACK	Amount	Cal.	Fat gm	Carb. gm	Fiber gm	Net Carb. gm	Protein gm
🕒 TOTAL							

LUNCH	Amount	Cal.	Fat gm	Carb. gm	Fiber gm	Net Carb. gm	Protein gm
🕒 TOTAL							

SNACK	Amount	Cal.	Fat gm	Carb. gm	Fiber gm	Net Carb. gm	Protein gm
🕒 TOTAL							

        8 oz

Step 2 – Tracking Food

DINNER	Amount	Cal.	Fat gm	Carb. gm	Fiber gm	Net Carb. gm	Protein gm
🕒 TOTAL							

SNACK	Amount	Cal.	Fat gm	Carb. gm	Fiber gm	Net Carb. gm	Protein gm
🕒 TOTAL							

| Daily Total | | | | | | | |
| Daily Target | | | | | | | |

Ketone Levels (mM)

|—|—|—|—|—|—|—|
0   0.5   1.0   1.5   2.0   2.5   3.0   5.0+

Fasting Clock

Fast start _____

Fast finish _____

Hours fasted [ ]

Exercise notes

What _____

Duration _____

Calories Burned _____

Vitamins / Supplements / Meds.

Description	Qty

How was today?

_____

_____

DAILY

Date: _____   Mon. Tue. Wed. Thur. Fri. Sat. Sun.

BREAKFAST	Amount	Cal.	Fat gm	Carb. gm	Fiber gm	Net Carb. gm	Protein gm
🕐 TOTAL							

SNACK	Amount	Cal.	Fat gm	Carb. gm	Fiber gm	Net Carb. gm	Protein gm
🕐 TOTAL							

LUNCH	Amount	Cal.	Fat gm	Carb. gm	Fiber gm	Net Carb. gm	Protein gm
🕐 TOTAL							

SNACK	Amount	Cal.	Fat gm	Carb. gm	Fiber gm	Net Carb. gm	Protein gm
🕐 TOTAL							

        8 oz

Step 2 – Tracking Food

DINNER	Amount	Cal.	Fat gm	Carb. gm	Fiber gm	Net Carb. gm	Protein gm
TOTAL							

SNACK	Amount	Cal.	Fat gm	Carb. gm	Fiber gm	Net Carb. gm	Protein gm
TOTAL							
Daily Total							
Daily Target							

Ketone Levels (mM)

0   0.5   1.0   1.5   2.0   2.5   3.0   5.0+

Fasting Clock

Fast start _____

Fast finish _____

Hours fasted

Exercise notes

What _____

Duration _____

Calories Burned _____

Vitamins / Supplements / Meds.

Description	Qty

How was today?

_____

_____

_____

DAILY

Date: _____   Mon. Tue. Wed. Thur. Fri. Sat. Sun.

BREAKFAST	Amount	Cal.	Fat gm	Carb. gm	Fiber gm	Net Carb. gm	Protein gm
🕒 TOTAL							

SNACK	Amount	Cal.	Fat gm	Carb. gm	Fiber gm	Net Carb. gm	Protein gm
🕒 TOTAL							

LUNCH	Amount	Cal.	Fat gm	Carb. gm	Fiber gm	Net Carb. gm	Protein gm
🕒 TOTAL							

SNACK	Amount	Cal.	Fat gm	Carb. gm	Fiber gm	Net Carb. gm	Protein gm
🕒 TOTAL							

8 oz

Step 2 – Tracking Food

DINNER	Amount	Cal.	Fat gm	Carb. gm	Fiber gm	Net Carb. gm	Protein gm
⏲ TOTAL							

SNACK	Amount	Cal.	Fat gm	Carb. gm	Fiber gm	Net Carb. gm	Protein gm
⏲ TOTAL							

| Daily Total | | | | | | | |
| Daily Target | | | | | | | |

Ketone Levels (mM)

|—|—|—|—|—|—|—|
0   0.5   1.0   1.5   2.0   2.5   3.0   5.0+

Fasting Clock

Fast start _____   Hours fasted

Fast finish _____

Exercise notes

What _____

Duration _____

Calories Burned _____

Vitamins / Supplements / Meds.

Description	Qty

How was today?

_____

_____

DAILY

Date: _____ Mon. Tue. Wed. Thur. Fri. Sat. Sun.

BREAKFAST	Amount	Cal.	Fat gm	Carb. gm	Fiber gm	Net Carb. gm	Protein gm
🕐 TOTAL							

SNACK	Amount	Cal.	Fat gm	Carb. gm	Fiber gm	Net Carb. gm	Protein gm
🕐 TOTAL							

LUNCH	Amount	Cal.	Fat gm	Carb. gm	Fiber gm	Net Carb. gm	Protein gm
🕐 TOTAL							

SNACK	Amount	Cal.	Fat gm	Carb. gm	Fiber gm	Net Carb. gm	Protein gm
🕐 TOTAL							

        8 oz

Step 2 – Tracking Food

DINNER	Amount	Cal.	Fat gm	Carb. gm	Fiber gm	Net Carb. gm	Protein gm
TOTAL							

SNACK	Amount	Cal.	Fat gm	Carb. gm	Fiber gm	Net Carb. gm	Protein gm
TOTAL							
Daily Total							
Daily Target							

Ketone Levels (mM)

|—|—|—|—|—|—|—|
0   0.5   1.0   1.5   2.0   2.5   3.0   5.0+

Fasting Clock

Fast start _____   Hours fasted

Fast finish _____

Exercise notes

What _____

Duration _____

Calories Burned _____

Vitamins / Supplements / Meds.

Description	Qty

How was today?

_____

_____

DAILY

Date: _____ Mon. Tue. Wed. Thur. Fri. Sat. Sun.

BREAKFAST	Amount	Cal.	Fat gm	Carb. gm	Fiber gm	Net Carb. gm	Protein gm
🕘 TOTAL							

SNACK	Amount	Cal.	Fat gm	Carb. gm	Fiber gm	Net Carb. gm	Protein gm
🕘 TOTAL							

LUNCH	Amount	Cal.	Fat gm	Carb. gm	Fiber gm	Net Carb. gm	Protein gm
🕘 TOTAL							

SNACK	Amount	Cal.	Fat gm	Carb. gm	Fiber gm	Net Carb. gm	Protein gm
🕘 TOTAL							

        8 oz

Step 2 – Tracking Food

DINNER	Amount	Cal.	Fat gm	Carb. gm	Fiber gm	Net Carb. gm	Protein gm
🕓 TOTAL							

SNACK	Amount	Cal.	Fat gm	Carb. gm	Fiber gm	Net Carb. gm	Protein gm
🕓 TOTAL							

| Daily Total | | | | | | | |
| Daily Target | | | | | | | |

Ketone Levels (mM)

|—|—|—|—|—|—|—|
0   0.5   1.0   1.5   2.0   2.5   3.0   5.0+

Fasting Clock

Fast start _____   Hours fasted

Fast finish _____

Exercise notes

What _____

Duration _____

Calories Burned _____

Vitamins / Supplements / Meds.

Description	Qty

How was today?

_____

_____

DAILY

Date: _____   Mon. Tue. Wed. Thur. Fri. Sat. Sun.

BREAKFAST	Amount	Cal.	Fat gm	Carb. gm	Fiber gm	Net Carb. gm	Protein gm
🕐 TOTAL							

SNACK	Amount	Cal.	Fat gm	Carb. gm	Fiber gm	Net Carb. gm	Protein gm
🕐 TOTAL							

LUNCH	Amount	Cal.	Fat gm	Carb. gm	Fiber gm	Net Carb. gm	Protein gm
🕐 TOTAL							

SNACK	Amount	Cal.	Fat gm	Carb. gm	Fiber gm	Net Carb. gm	Protein gm
🕐 TOTAL							

        8 oz

Step 2 – Tracking Food

DINNER	Amount	Cal.	Fat gm	Carb. gm	Fiber gm	Net Carb. gm	Protein gm
TOTAL							

SNACK	Amount	Cal.	Fat gm	Carb. gm	Fiber gm	Net Carb. gm	Protein gm
TOTAL							

Daily Total							
Daily Target							

Ketone Levels (mM)
0   0.5   1.0   1.5   2.0   2.5   3.0   5.0+

Fasting Clock
Fast start _____   Hours fasted
Fast finish _____

Exercise notes
What _____
Duration _____
Calories Burned _____

Vitamins / Supplements / Meds.

Description	Qty

How was today?
_____
_____

"**IT'S NOT A SHORT TERM DIET, IT'S A LONG TERM LIFESTYLE CHANGE**"

STEP 3
REVIEW

Reviewing your progress keeps you motivated. It shows how far you have come and encourages you to keep going when it gets hard.

In this section you can record your vital statistics across time as well as before and after measurements.

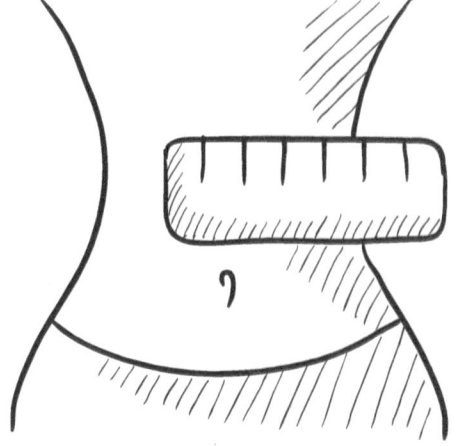

BEFORE AND AFTER

Record your before-and-after statistics to see how far you have come. Record as many or as few as you like.

Set the date for the before and after. We'd recommend three months from now, which is one cycle of the journal.

There are blank rows if you want to track anything specific.

	BEFORE	AFTER	CHANGE	GOAL
Date	Jan. 1st	Mar. 30th		
Weight	180lbs	160lbs	-20lbs	165lbs
Blood pressure				
Cholesterol level				
Body measurements				
Neck				
Arms				
Chest				
Waist	42 inches	36 inches	-4 inches	2 inches
Hips				
Thighs				
Dress size	16	14	1 size	1 size

Tips:

- Measure yourself in the morning before any food or water. Be consistent with each measurement.
- Be realistic about your goals.

Step 3 – Review

	BEFORE	AFTER	CHANGE	GOAL
Date				
Weight				
Blood pressure				
Cholesterol level				
Body measurements				
Neck				
Arms				
Chest				
Waist				
Hips				
Thighs				

TRACKING CHARTS

Use the below chart to track your cumulative weight-loss across the weeks. Seeing your progress on the chart shows how far you have come and keeps you motivated.

Use either dates (e.g. January 1st) or days (e.g. day 1, day 2 etc) along the bottom and your own scale along the side (e.g. starting at 180lbs and using 2lb increments). Measure your weight as frequently as you feel comfortable with. Some people like the accountability of measuring every day, whilst others find it stressful. It is recommended that you measure at least once a week.

The charts can also be used for tracking other metrics. Perhaps track your ketone levels, calories per day, exercise levels, such as minutes per day walked or your mood – based on a five-point scale. This is all optional but have some fun with it.

Step 3 – Review

WEEKLY PROGRESS CHART

	Week 1	Week 2	Week 3	Week 4	Week 5	Week 6	Week 7	Week 8	Week 9	Week 10	Week 11	Week 12
Weight - Actual	180	175	173	171	170	168	166	166	164	162	160	160
Weight - Change		5	2	2	1	2	2	0	2	2	2	0
Blood Pressure												
Cholesterol Level												
Body Measurements												
Neck												
Arms												
Chest												
Waist	42	40	39.5	39	38.5	38	37.5	37.5	37	36.5	36	36
Hips												
Thighs												

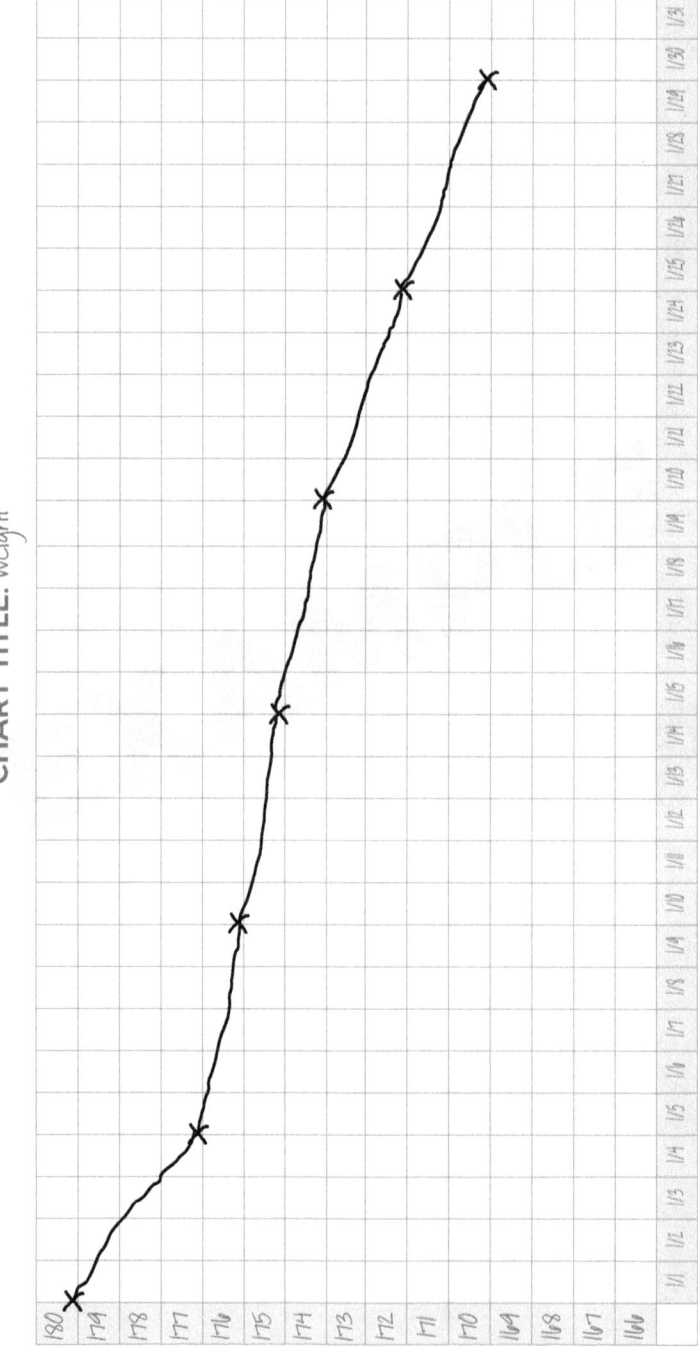

Step 3 – Review

WEEKLY PROGRESS CHART

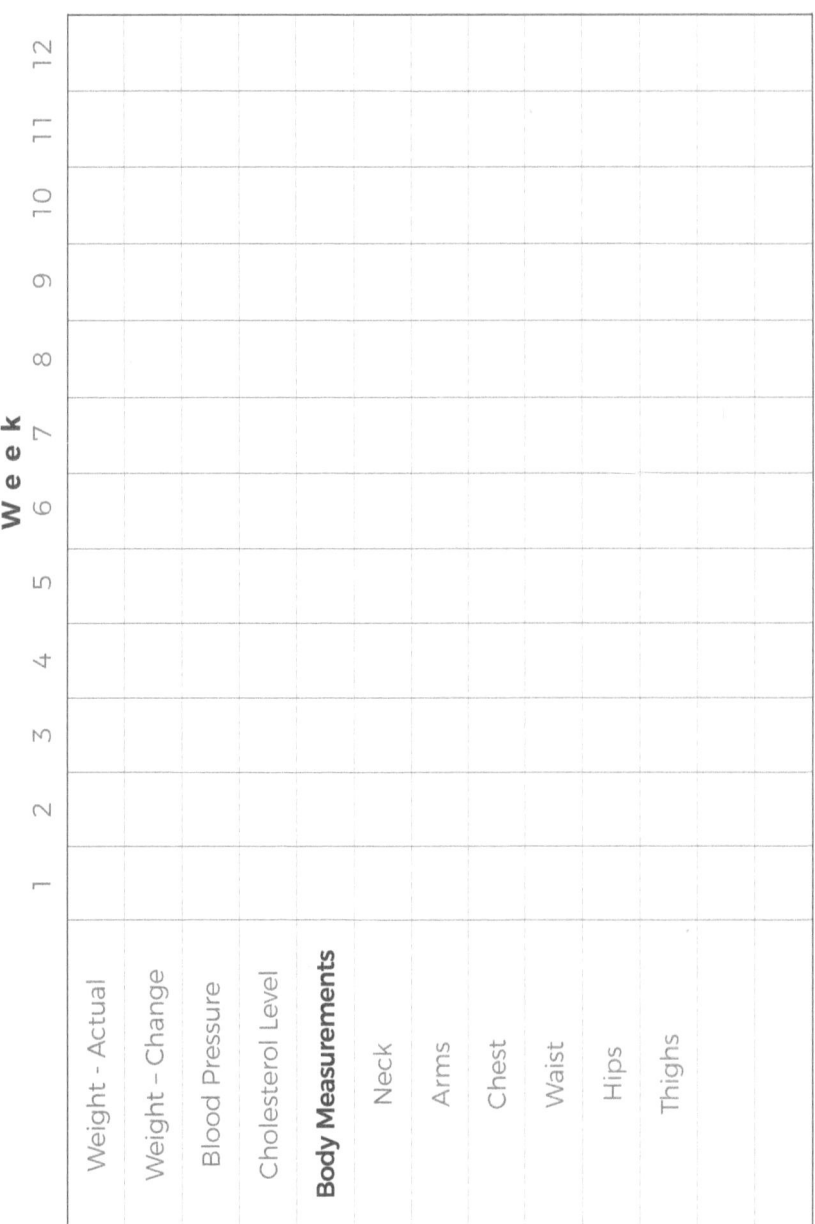

CHART TITLE:

RANGE

DATE / DAY

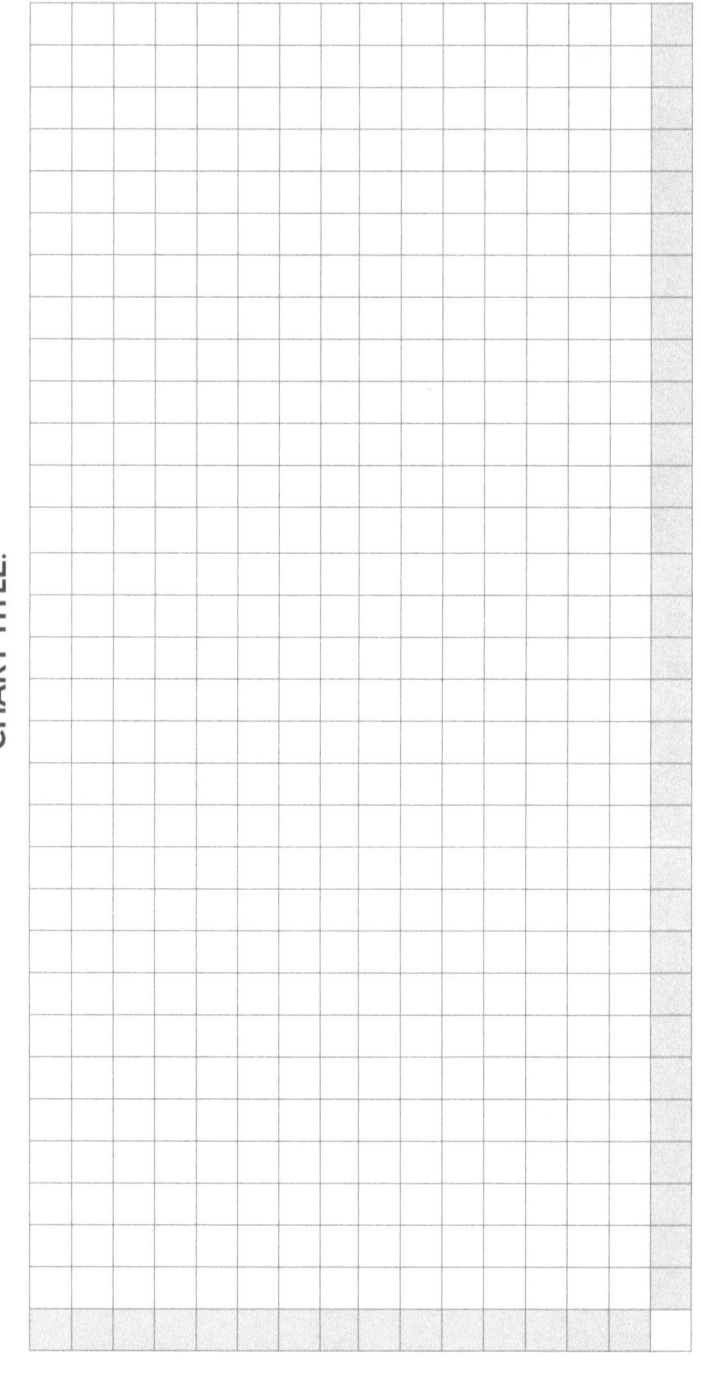

CHART TITLE:

DATE / DAY

RANGE

STEP 4
CELEBRATE

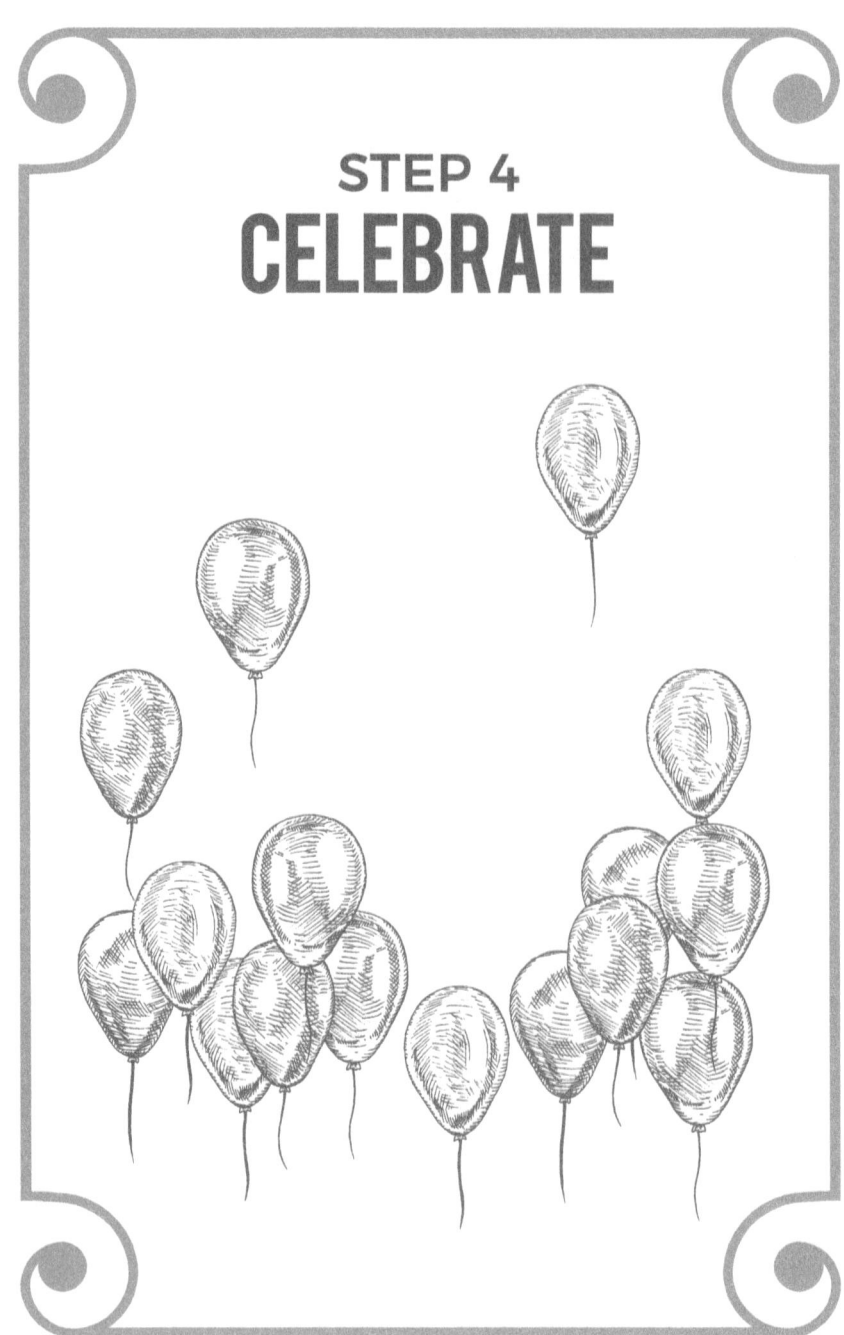

3-MONTH TARGET ACHIEVED

Congratulations – you have achieved three months of tracking your nutrition and working toward your goals. It is definitely time to celebrate.

Whether or not you have achieved your exact goals or have just made progress toward them, I want to sincerely congratulate you and wish you the best for the next steps.

I would invite you to review your journey during the past three months.

- What have you achieved?
- What patterns have emerged?
- What old habits did you have that you can now avoid?
- How can you reinforce your new habits?

I would also love to hear your story and feedback on the process. Please email us at help@habitually-healthy.com and bring a little smile to our faces ☺

Habitually Healthy

Deluxe Keto & Low Carb Food Journal

> **"IT DOESN'T MATTER HOW FAST OR SLOWLY YOU, SO LONG AS YOU DO NOT STOP"**

APPENDIX

There are several useful reference guides and templates to make the journey easier. Inside you will find:

- Common daily activities and calories burned (some may surprise you).

- A template to record your frequently eaten meals (for easy nutritional reference)

- Recipe notes templates to record your favorite recipes (including ingredients, directions and more)

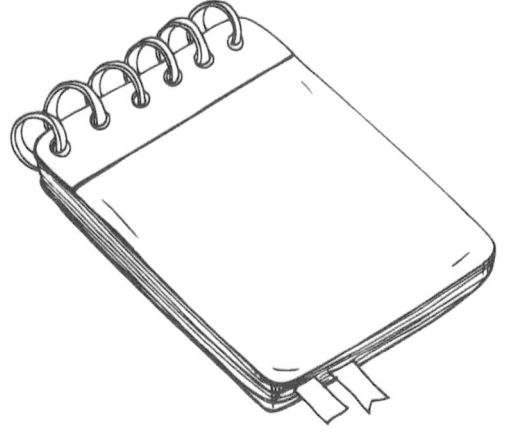

EXERCISE REFERENCE GUIDE

Actual calories burned will vary person to person, dependent on age, gender, metabolism, height, and weight. However, below is a handy list of calories burnt for 30 minutes of activity.

Calories burned in 30-minute activities	
Gym Activities	185-pound person
Aerobics: water	178
Stretching, Hatha yoga	178
Aerobics: low impact	244
Steeper machine: general	266
Aerobics, step: low impact	311
Bicycling, stationary: moderate	311
Rowing, stationary: moderate	311
Training and Sport Activities	
Badminton: general	200
Basketball: general play	355
Bicycling: 12-13.9 mph	355
Dancing: slow, waltz, foxtrot	133
Hiking: cross-country	266
Rope: jumping	444
Running: 5 mph (12 min./mile)	355
Running: 7.5 mph (8 min/mile)	555

Running: 7.5 mph (8 min/mile)	555
Soccer: general	311
Softball: general play	222
Swimming: general	266
Tennis: general	311
Walk/jog: jog <10 min	266
Walking: 4 mph (15 min./mile)	200
Outdoor Activities	
Raking lawn	178
Sacking grass or leaves	178
Gardening: general	200
Dancing: slow, waltz, foxtrot	200
Mowing lawn: push, power	200
Laying sod / crushed rock	222
Mowing lawn: push, hand	244
Home and Daily Life Activities	
Playing with kids: moderate effort	178
Heavy cleaning: wash car, windows	200
Child games: hopscotch, jacks	222
Playing with kids: vigorous effort	222
Moving: household furniture	266
Moving: carrying boxes	311

FREQUENTLY EATEN FOODS

Record your favorite meals for easy reference.

MEALS	Amount	Cal.	Fat gm	Carb. gm	Fiber gm	Net Carb. gm	Protein gm
Avo' Burger	1 burger	232	20			3	10
Breakfast smoothie	1 glass	178	14			1	12

FREQUENTLY EATEN FOODS

MEALS	Amount	Cal.	Fat gm	Carb. gm	Fiber gm	Net Carb. gm	Protein gm

Deluxe Keto & Low Carb Food Journal

RECIPE NOTES

Use this space to record any new favorite recipes you find.

Recipe Name

Ingredients

-
-
-
-
-
-
-
-

Directions

Recommended Occasions

Notes

RECIPE #

Where is the recipe from?

Serves
1 2 3 4 5 6

Prep Time :
Cook Time :

Prep Type

Goes Well With

Nutritional Info
Calories
Fat
Carb
Fiber
Net Carb
Protein

How Tasty?
Difficulty:
1 2 3 4 5
Overall Rating:

Appendix

RECIPE NOTES

Use this space to record any new favorite recipes you find.

Recipe Name

_____

Ingredients
- _____   • _____
- _____   • _____
- _____   • _____
- _____   • _____
- _____   • _____
- _____   • _____

Directions

_____
_____
_____
_____
_____
_____
_____
_____

Recommended Occasions

_____
_____

Notes

_____
_____
_____

RECIPE #

Where is the recipe from?

_____

Serves
1   2   3   4   5   6

Prep Time : _____
Cook Time : _____

Prep Type

_____
_____

Goes Well With

_____
_____

Nutritional Info
Calories   _____
Fat   _____
Carb   _____
Fiber   _____
Net Carb   _____
Protein   _____

How Tasty?
Difficulty:
1   2   3   4   5
Overall Rating:
☹ 😕 😐 🙂 😄

Deluxe Keto & Low Carb Food Journal

RECIPE NOTES

Use this space to record any new favorite recipes you find.

Recipe Name

RECIPE #

Ingredients

- _____
- _____
- _____
- _____
- _____
- _____
- _____
- _____
- _____
- _____

Where is the recipe from?
_____

Serves
1 2 3 4 5 6

Prep Time :_____
Cook Time :_____

Directions

Prep Type
_____
_____

Goes Well With
_____
_____

Nutritional Info
Calories _____
Fat   _____
Carb   _____
Fiber   _____
Net Carb _____
Protein   _____

Recommended Occasions

Notes

How Tasty?
Difficulty:
1 2 3 4 5
Overall Rating:
😖 😒 😐 🙂 😄

Appendix

RECIPE NOTES

Use this space to record any new favorite recipes you find.

Recipe Name

_____

Ingredients

- _____
- _____
- _____
- _____
- _____
- _____
- _____
- _____
- _____
- _____

Directions

_____
_____
_____
_____
_____
_____
_____
_____
_____
_____

Recommended Occasions

_____
_____

Notes

_____
_____
_____

RECIPE #

Where is the recipe from?

_____

Serves
1 2 3 4 5 6

Prep Time : _____
Cook Time : _____

Prep Type

_____
_____

Goes Well With

_____
_____

Nutritional Info
Calories _____
Fat   _____
Carb   _____
Fiber   _____
Net Carb _____
Protein   _____

How Tasty?
Difficulty:
1 2 3 4 5
Overall Rating:
😞 😕 😐 😊 😁

RECIPE NOTES

Use this space to record any new favorite recipes you find.

Recipe Name

_____

Ingredients
- _____ • _____
- _____ • _____
- _____ • _____
- _____ • _____
- _____ • _____

Directions

_____
_____
_____
_____
_____
_____
_____
_____

Recommended Occasions

_____
_____

Notes

_____
_____
_____

RECIPE #

Where is the recipe from?
_____

Serves
1   2   3   4   5   6

Prep Time : _____
Cook Time : _____

Prep Type
_____
_____

Goes Well With
_____
_____

Nutritional Info
Calories _____
Fat   _____
Carb   _____
Fiber   _____
Net Carb _____
Protein   _____

How Tasty?
Difficulty:
1   2   3   4   5
Overall Rating:
😟 😔 😐 🙂 😄

Appendix

RECIPE NOTES

Use this space to record any new favorite recipes you find.

Recipe Name

_____

RECIPE #

Ingredients

- _____
- _____
- _____
- _____
- _____
- _____
- _____
- _____
- _____
- _____

Where is the recipe from?

_____

Serves
1   2   3   4   5   6

Prep Time : _____
Cook Time : _____

Directions

_____
_____
_____
_____
_____
_____
_____
_____
_____
_____
_____
_____

Prep Type

_____
_____

Goes Well With

_____
_____

Nutritional Info
Calories _____
Fat   _____
Carb   _____
Fiber   _____
Net Carb _____
Protein   _____

Recommended Occasions

_____
_____

Notes

_____
_____
_____

How Tasty?
Difficulty:
1   2   3   4   5
Overall Rating:
😖 😒 😐 🙂 😄

Deluxe Keto & Low Carb Food Journal

RECIPE NOTES

Use this space to record any new favorite recipes you find.

Recipe Name

RECIPE #

Ingredients

-
-
-
-
-
-
-
-
-
-

Where is the recipe from?

Serves
1   2   3   4   5   6

Prep Time :
Cook Time :

Directions

Prep Type

Goes Well With

Nutritional Info
Calories
Fat
Carb
Fiber
Net Carb
Protein

Recommended Occasions

How Tasty?
Difficulty:
1   2   3   4   5
Overall Rating:

Notes

Appendix

RECIPE NOTES

Use this space to record any new favorite recipes you find.

Recipe Name

Ingredients
- _____   • _____
- _____   • _____
- _____   • _____
- _____   • _____
- _____   • _____
- _____   • _____

Directions

_____

_____

_____

_____

_____

_____

_____

_____

Recommended Occasions

_____

_____

Notes

_____

_____

_____

RECIPE #

Where is the recipe from?

_____

Serves
1   2   3   4   5   6

Prep Time : _____
Cook Time : _____

Prep Type

_____

Goes Well With

_____

_____

Nutritional Info
Calories _____
Fat   _____
Carb   _____
Fiber   _____
Net Carb _____
Protein   _____

How Tasty?
Difficulty:
1   2   3   4   5
Overall Rating:
😟 😕 😐 🙂 😁

RECIPE NOTES

Use this space to record any new favorite recipes you find.

Recipe Name

_____

Ingredients
- _____
- _____
- _____
- _____
- _____
- _____
- _____
- _____
- _____
- _____

Directions

_____
_____
_____
_____
_____
_____
_____
_____
_____

Recommended Occasions

_____
_____

Notes

_____
_____
_____

RECIPE #

Where is the recipe from?
_____

Serves
1 2 3 4 5 6

Prep Time : _____
Cook Time : _____

Prep Type
_____
_____

Goes Well With
_____
_____

Nutritional Info
Calories _____
Fat _____
Carb _____
Fiber _____
Net Carb _____
Protein _____

How Tasty?
Difficulty:
1 2 3 4 5
Overall Rating:
😖 😕 😐 🙂 😄

Appendix

RECIPE NOTES

Use this space to record any new favorite recipes you find.

Recipe Name

Ingredients
- _____
- _____
- _____
- _____
- _____
- _____

Directions

Recommended Occasions

Notes

RECIPE #

Where is the recipe from?

Serves
1   2   3   4   5   6

Prep Time :_____
Cook Time :_____

Prep Type

Goes Well With

Nutritional Info
Calories _____
Fat _____
Carb _____
Fiber _____
Net Carb _____
Protein _____

How Tasty?
Difficulty:
1   2   3   4   5
Overall Rating:
😟 😕 😐 🙂 😄

Deluxe Keto & Low Carb Food Journal

RECIPE NOTES

Use this space to record any new favorite recipes you find.

Recipe Name

RECIPE #

Ingredients

Where is the recipe from?

-
-
-
-
-
-

Serves
1   2   3   4   5   6

Prep Time :
Cook Time :

Directions

Prep Type

Goes Well With

Nutritional Info
Calories
Fat
Carb
Fiber

Recommended Occasions

Net Carb
Protein

How Tasty?
Difficulty:
1   2   3   4   5

Notes

Overall Rating:

254

Appendix

RECIPE NOTES

Use this space to record any new favorite recipes you find.

Recipe Name
_____

Ingredients
- _____
- _____
- _____
- _____
- _____
- _____
- _____
- _____
- _____
- _____

Directions
_____
_____
_____
_____
_____
_____
_____
_____

Recommended Occasions
_____
_____

Notes
_____
_____
_____

RECIPE #

Where is the recipe from?
_____

Serves
1   2   3   4   5   6

Prep Time : _____
Cook Time : _____

Prep Type
_____
_____

Goes Well With
_____
_____

Nutritional Info
Calories   _____
Fat   _____
Carb   _____
Fiber   _____
Net Carb   _____
Protein   _____

How Tasty?
Difficulty:
1   2   3   4   5
Overall Rating:
😟 😒 😐 😊 😄

www.ingramcontent.com/pod-product-compliance
Lightning Source LLC
Chambersburg PA
CBHW020108240426
43661CB00002B/71